INTERVENTIONAL
BREAST
PROCEDURES

INTERVENTIONAL BREAST PROCEDURES

Edited by

D. David Dershaw, M.D.
Director
Breast Imaging Section
Department of Radiology
Memorial Sloan-Kettering Cancer Center
Associate Professor
Department of Radiology
Cornell University Medical College
New York, New York

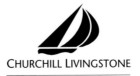

CHURCHILL LIVINGSTONE

New York, Edinburgh, London, Madrid, Melbourne, San Francisco, Tokyo

Library of Congress Cataloging-in-Publication Data

Distributed in the United Kingdom by Churchill Livingstone, Robert Stevenson House, 1–3 Baxter's Place, Leith Walk, Edinburgh EH1 3AF, and by associated companies, branches, and representatives throughout the world.

Accurate indications, adverse reactions, and dosage schedules for drugs are provided in this book, but it is possible that they may change. The reader is urged to review the pack-age information data of the manufacturers of the medications mentioned.

The Publishers have made every effort to trace the copyright holders for borrowed mate-rial. If they have inadvertently overlooked any, they will be pleased to make the neces-sary arrangements at the first opportunity.

Acquisitions Editors: *Miranda Bromage and Michael J. Houston*
Production Editor: *Dorothy J. Birch*
Production Supervisor: *Laura Mosberg Cohen*
Desktop Coordinator: *Jo-Ann Demas*
Cover Design: *Paul Moran*

Printed in the United States of America

First published in 1996   7   6   5   4   3   2   1

*To honor Lucille and Samuel
and for Beckie and Bruce*

CONTRIBUTORS

R. James Brenner, M.D., J.D.

Associate Professor, Department of Radiology, University of California, Los Angeles, UCLA School of Medicine, Los Angeles, California; Director, Breast Imaging Services, Eisenberg Keefer Breast Center, John Wayne Cancer Institute, Santa Monica, California

Gilda Cardenosa, M.D.

Associate Professor, Department of Radiology, University of Illinois College of Medicine at Peoria; Medical Director, Susan G. Komen Breast Center, St. Francis Medical Center, Peoria, Illinois

Ellen Shaw de Paredes, M.D.

Professor, Division of Diagnostic Radiology, Department of Radiology, Virginia Commonwealth University Medical College of Virginia School of Medicine; Director, Breast Imaging, Department of Radiology, Medical College of Virginia Hospitals, Richmond, Virginia

D. David Dershaw, M.D.

Associate Professor, Department of Radiology, Cornell University Medical College; Director, Breast Imaging Section, Department of Radiology, Memorial Sloan-Kettering Cancer Center, New York, New York

G. W. Eklund, M.D.

Professor, Department of Radiology, University of Illinois College of Medicine at Peoria; Staff Physician, Susan G. Komen Breast Center, St. Francis Medical Center, Peoria, Illinois

W. Phil Evans, M.D.

Associate Professor, Department of Radiology, University of Texas Southwestern Medical Center at Dallas Southwestern Medical School; Medical Director, Susan G. Komen Breast Center, Baylor University Medical Center, Dallas, Texas

Laurie Farjado, M.D.

Associate Professor and Vice Chairman of Research, Department of Radiology, University of Virginia School of Medicine; Radiologist, Department of Radiology, University of Virginia Hospital, Charlottesville, Virginia

David P. Gorczyca, M.D.

Assistant Professor, Iris Cantor Center for Breast Imaging, Department of Radiological Sciences, University of California, Los Angeles, UCLA School of Medicine, Los Angeles, California; Radiologist, Department of Radiology, Sunrise Hospital Medical Center, Las Vegas, Nevada

Debra M. Ikeda, M.D.

Assistant Professor, Department of Radiology, Stanford University School of Medicine; Section Chief, Division of Breast Imaging, Department of Radiology, Stanford University Hospital, Stanford, California

Laura Liberman, M.D.

Assistant Professor, Department of Radiology, Cornell University Medical College; Assistant Attending Physician, Department of Radiology, Memorial Sloan-Kettering Cancer Center, New York, New York

Ellen B. Mendelson, M.D.

Associate Professor, Division of Diagnostic Radiology, Department of Radiology, University of Pittsburgh School of Medicine; Director, Mammography and Women's Imaging, Department of Radiology, Western Pennsylvania Hospital, Pittsburgh, Pennsylvania

Etta D. Pisano, M.D.

Associate Professor, Department of Radiology, University of North Carolina at Chapel Hill School of Medicine; Director, Breast Imaging, University of North Carolina Hospitals, Chapel Hill, North Carolina

Paul Peter Rosen, M.D.

Professor, Department of Pathology, Cornell University Medical College; Attending Pathologist, Department of Pathology, Memorial Sloan-Kettering Cancer Center, New York, New York

Bruce J. Youngson, M.D.

Assistant Professor, Department of Pathology, University of Toronto Faculty of Medicine; Staff Pathologist, Department of Pathology, The Toronto Hospital, Toronto, Ontario, Canada

PREFACE

The role of the radiologist in the diagnosis and treatment of breast diseases has dramatically expanded in the past decade. It has become our responsibility not only to diagnose early cancers and characterize clinically evident disease but also to perform procedures that will often eliminate the need for surgical intervention. Some radiologists have sought to avoid these procedures that are increasingly a part of breast imaging. They may be untrained in these procedures or unfamiliar with the techniques necessary to perform them. Other radiologists are uncertain about the indications or contraindications for these procedures. *Interventional Breast Procedures* has been written to help in the selection of patients for these procedures and in the performance of these interventions. It is also designed to help the physician who may not be familiar with breast pathology to interpret the results of biopsy procedures and determine how they should be used in patient management. Legal issues involved in interventional breast procedures are also addressed.

Multiple authors have contributed to this text, representing many of the most prominent radiologists in the United States who have written about and performed the procedures described within these pages. Not surprisingly, some diversity of opinions is also present within this book. Rather than presenting the reader with a single perspective on some of the issues that surround interventional breast procedures, it was felt that this diversity would more honestly represent the status of these procedures.

It is hoped that this book will encourage radiologists to provide more comprehensive care to women with breast diseases. It is designed as a "how to" book with a practical discussion of all the invasive breast procedures that should be part of a breast radiologist's skills. The contributors to *Interventional Breast Procedures* hope that this book will make these procedures easier to understand and perform, and therefore more readily incorporated into the practice of all radiologists involved in breast imaging.

D. David Dershaw, M.D.

INTRODUCTION

The need for a book on interventional breast procedures results from a remarkable metamorphosis that the field of breast imaging has undergone since its inception. It was over three decades ago that radiologists first began to make radiographic images of the breast and concluded that there was clinical utility in these images. Following these events, it took years for surgeons to understand that breast cancer could be diagnosed mammographically before it was evident on physical examination and that early diagnosis would result in increased patient survival; when this happened, the era of screening mammography began. Although the battle over the application of mammography for screening is still being waged in some quarters, breast imaging has expanded from primitive radiographic examinations to studies that are now performed with highly specialized equipment; sonography and magnetic resonance imaging, as well as radiographic studies, are now within the domain of breast radiologists.

Because of the widespread application of breast imaging, especially screening mammography, a need has developed to assess breast lesions that are nonspecific to determine if they require therapeutic surgery. The discovery of nonpalpable, suspicious lesions on mammography has led to the development of needle localization procedures to pinpoint areas of suspected pathology that will be surgically removed. At the same time the widening application of breast conserving surgical techniques with the resultant awareness of the need to treat breast cancer by removing as little breast tissue as possible has promoted the development of procedures to diagnose lesions without surgical biopsy. Percutaneous breast biopsy techniques have been developed to meet this need. Finally, in the United States as well as in other nations, the growing awareness of the need to limit the cost of health care has helped to promote new, less expensive options for diagnosis that do not compromise quality of care. These circumstances have promoted the utilization of interventional breast procedures, performed by the radiologist, for the diagnosis of nonpalpable, and on occasion palpable, lesions within the breast. These procedures are performed quickly, with minimal trauma, without resulting deformity, in significantly less time, and with a considerable decrease in expense when compared to traditional surgical biopsy. Because of the importance of sonography in the assessment of breast disease and the growing importance of magnetic resonance imaging in breast imaging, techniques that allow localization of lesions and percutaneous biopsy with these imaging modalities have also been developed.

The breast imaging radiologist must have direct patient contact unlike the standard radiology practice in which the patient is often not directly in contact with the radiologist. In addition to the need for direct patient contact when the results of imaging studies are communicated, the performance of interventional studies also brings the radiologist into direct patient contact. While this book is designed to assist the radiologist in performing interventional procedures that have become an integral part of breast imaging, it cannot be overemphasized that all of these procedures need to be done with an understanding of the fear with which patients approach these interventions. The anxiety attendant on these studies is based not only on the pain that may accompany the procedure but also on the discovery of cancer that may result from it. Therefore, compassion is an essential part of performing any of these procedures. Before any of these procedures are done, they should be fully explained to the patient, and she should be treated with gentleness and understanding during the procedure.

The radiologist must also appreciate that the technologist is a partner to the physician when these procedures are undertaken. The emotional support given by the technologist to the patient before, during, and after the procedures is essential to patient cooperation and satisfaction. The technologists who are most successful in assisting with these procedures often combine the skills of technologists trained in mammography, sonography, and interventional radiology. It is important that physicians appreciate the special skills and accomplishments of technologists who can successfully assist during these procedures.

For the radiologist who is performing percutaneous biopsy procedures, an understanding of the significance of the results of the biopsy is also necessary. The responsibility for interpreting the clinical implications of the biopsy result lies with the physician who performed the tissue sampling. Radiologists who do breast biopsies must be able to determine whether the lesion in question has in fact been biopsied, whether the pathologic results are appropriate for the imaging characteristics of the lesion, and whether the entity diagnosed requires wider surgical excision to assess for a possible coexistent carcinoma. A thorough understanding of the imaging characteristics of the spectrum of breast disease is therefore needed to adequately evaluate whether or not the histology report is appropriate for the lesion that has undergone biopsy. A system for communicating results to the patient must be established. This may entail informing the referring clinician of the biopsy results, or the radiologist who performs the biopsy may directly communicate these results to the patient. In the latter situation, the radiologist who performs the biopsy must feel comfortable with this task and with arranging for appropriate treatment, if necessary. Again, significant patient interaction is required in these tasks, and the radiologist must be comfortable with these interactions.

As with all interventional procedures, those involving the breast include a certain risk of complication. Both the radiologist and the woman undergoing the procedure must be aware of these risks. Additionally, the radiologist must be prepared to have these complications treated. He or she must also be aware of the legal implications inherent in performing any of these procedures before they are undertaken.

Many of the procedures discussed in this book are performed in conjunction with our surgical colleagues. For example, needle localization and ductography are designed to assist surgeons as they search for or remove lesions. Percutaneous breast biopsy procedures, however, have become a source of confrontation in some practices. Is it necessary that these procedures be performed by a radiologist or can they be done with equal competence by a surgeon or other physician? Do radiologists possess the special training necessary to do these procedures? These questions are moot when biopsies are done under sonographic guidance. Surgeons have no pretense of competence in this highly operator dependent modality. The special training needed to perform these procedures and possessed by radiologists is self-evident. The same will be true of biopsy procedures performed with magnetic resonance imaging guidance, when this technology becomes more widely available. When biopsies are done under stereotaxic imaging, however, nonradiologists sometimes feel that special competence in imaging is not necessary. It is undoubtedly true that many times these biopsies are easily performed with the user-friendly equipment that is now available. However, not all lesions are readily discernible on the small field of view available during stereotaxic procedures. It may be difficult to localize the lesion, to identify the same calcification on the stereo pairs, and to adjust the image so that subtle tissue differences can be appreciated. It may require significant skill in understanding how two two-dimensional images reflect the geometry of a three-dimensional structure so that the patient can be appropriately positioned to accommodate the depth needed for a cutting needle to move through the breast. These procedures also involve exposing a woman to radiation. Increased facility at performing these biopsies often results in a decreased number of images needed to successfully complete the procedure and therefore a decreased amount of radiation to which the woman is exposed during the biopsy. Because of these reasons, image-guided breast biopsy procedures should be performed by radiologists. Radiologists who are well trained to do these procedures will perform them with skills that our surgical colleagues have not needed to develop in their specialty.

This book has been organized to address the indications, contraindications, techniques, and patient care patterns that are appropriate to image-guided interventional breast procedures. This book does not suggest that all the authors contributing to this text or that all radiologists performing these procedures agree with the protocols outlined for each procedure. Controversy exists over the indication of pneumocystography as a procedure to prevent cysts from reforming. A variety of post-biospy protocols exist for the routine care of women who have undergone fine needle aspiration or large-core breast biopsy, and the utility of differing biopsy techniques (i.e., FNA versus core biopsy) remains controversial. The reader should understand that the methods of patient care described herein may be altered or modified to suit individual practices or individual patients. The reader should also notice that there is some overlapping material presented in some chapters. This will enable the reader to obtain a more comprehensive discussion of individual topics without needing to refer to multiple chapters. A more in-depth discussion of specific topics, however, is available in the chapters designed to address these specific issues.

It is my intent and the intent of my co-authors that this book aid and encourage those involved in breast imaging to undertake the procedures described here-in. Their widespread availability will improve the quality of breast care provided to women. Additionally, the incorporation of these procedures into a breast imaging practice will lead to a more comprehensive and satisfying practice.

Interventional Breast Procedures has been a collaborative effort, and I wish to express my appreciation to my colleagues and friends who have graciously agreed to contribute to it. This project would not have been successful, and in fact, I would not have undertaken it, without their willingness to partcipate. They have been generous in giving their time and energy toward this project. They represent many of the leading authorities in interventional breast procedures and the legal and histopathologic sequelae of these procedures. I am grateful for their willingness to share their expertise with me and with those who will read this book. It is our hope that this volume will aid radiologists in their continuing efforts to diagnose early breast cancers and enable women not only to be more readily cured of this disease, but to be treated in a more speedy and less disfiguring fashion.

D. David Dershaw, M.D.

CONTENTS

1 DUCTOGRAPHY

Gilda Cardenosa
G. W. Eklund

Spontaneous, unilateral, single duct discharge (bloody, serous, or clear) is the most common manifestation of solitary papillomas.[1,2] Fibrocystic change and duct ectasia can also present with spontaneous nipple discharge.[2] In these entities, however, the discharge commonly originates from multiple ducts bilaterally, is often nonspontaneous (expressed), and is either thick green in fibrocystic change or pasty white with duct ectasia. Spontaneous, single duct discharge, which is either bloody, serous, or clear, can occur in patients with breast cancer.[2–4] Clinically, most patients with spontaneous nipple discharge do not have an associated palpable abnormality; however, a "trigger point" can sometimes be identified.[5] Compression at the site of the underlying intraductal abnormality (the "trigger point") may elicit discharge.

Most patients with spontaneous nipple discharge have normal mammograms. Occasionally, a dilated duct (Fig. 1-1), which may have associated coarse calcifications, can be seen in patients with solitary papillomas. Ductography is the procedure of choice in evaluating patients with spontaneous nipple discharge.[4] When the abnormal duct is cannulated and contrast injected, the number, location, and extent of intraductal lesions can be demonstrated reliably. Because of high false-negative and false positive rates, exfoliative cytology of nipple discharge has no role in the evaluation and management of patients with spontaneous nipple discharge.[4]

Ductography is a safe and easy procedure. We routinely use a 30-gauge straight (1.5 cm), blunt tip, sialography needle (Ranfac, Avon, Massachusetts) connected to a luer hub at the end of a 30 cm clear tube. Also available are 30-gauge, blunt-tipped needles with a 90-degree bend. This angulation purportedly facilitates cannulation and helps anchor the needle within the duct. Undiluted iothalamate meglumine (Conray 60; Mallinckrodt, St. Louis) in a 3 cc luer lock syringe is run through the tubing and needle. Air bubbles are flushed out. Some authors recommend the use of nonionic contrast agents. We have had no complications using Conray 60, even in patients with a history of contrast allergy. The risk of reaction is minimized by the use of small amounts of contrast (0.2 to 0.4 cc) and intraductal rather than intravenous injection. In addition, most of the contrast is expressed or leaks out of the duct at the completion of the study.[6,7]

Patients can be sitting or supine. They are more relaxed and comfortable, however, in the supine position, which facilitates the identification and cannulation of the secreting duct orifice. At the onset, the nipple is wiped with alcohol. Because several duct openings are commonly clustered together on the surface of the nipple, it is important to spend some time identifying the discharging duct. If the discharge has been ongoing for several years, the duct opening may be slightly more prominent, erythematous, and

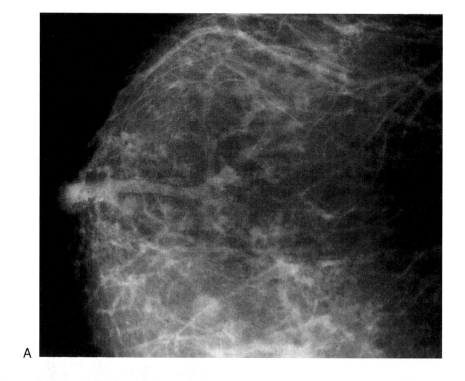

A

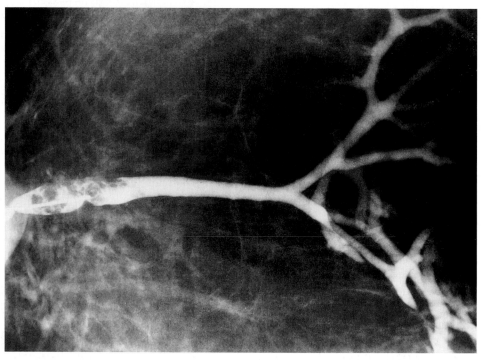

B

Fig. 1-1. (A) Screening mammogram in a patient with spontaneous nipple discharge demonstrates a single dilated duct. **(B)** An irregular filling defect is identified following opacification of the dilated duct seen mammographically. A papilloma was diagnosed histologically. (Magnification × 1.8)

patulous compared with adjacent openings. If a trigger point is found, it can be used to elicit tiny droplets of discharge at the ductal opening. The droplet can be wiped and additional droplets elicited as many times as needed to identify clearly the involved ductal orifice for cannulation. Adequate lighting focused on the nipple and magnification (using magnification lenses on a head mount or attached to prescription or safety glasses) expedite the procedure.

Inverted nipples can present a challenge. By applying pressure on the subareolar area or circumferential traction on the nipple/areola, the nipple can often be everted just enough to expose the ductal opening.[6,7]

After the offending ductal opening is identified, the tip of the cannula is gently placed in the orifice. Once engaged, the cannula often "falls" into the duct, usually to the hub. If the patient experiences pain when the cannula is engaged, or if force is needed to advance the cannula, it is best to stop to reassess needle placement accuracy. The tip of the cannula may be on a nipple crevice rather than in a duct. Some lesions are close to the nipple so that resistance or impediment to needle advancement may be encountered. In some patients, cannulation is prevented by nipple smooth muscle contraction around the duct orifices. A hot washcloth applied to the nipple helps relax the smooth muscle enough to permit cannulation. Alternatively, circumferential traction and lifting of the nipple (presumably straightening the course of the duct subareolarly) after the tip of the cannula is engaged in the ductal orifice are maneuvers that can be used to cannulate the duct and facilitate advancement of the cannula. Local anesthesia or ductal dilation is not needed.[6,7]

With the duct cannulated, the needle is secured in place with two pieces of paper tape, and contrast is injected slowly. It is advisable to start with 0.2 to 0.4 cc of contrast because small lesions may be obscured as more contrast is injected. If the patient complains of pain or burning, the injection is stopped and, with the needle still in place, full paddle magnified images in the craniocaudal and 90-degree lateral projections are obtained. Keeping the cannula in the duct minimizes reflux when compression is applied and permits injection of additional contrast if the initial images demonstrate inadequate ductal filling. After the procedure is completed the patient is given a pad (Curity Disposable Nursing Pads, The Kendall Co.,

Boston) to insert in her bra to protect her clothing from leaking contrast.[6,7]

Normal ducts have variable luminal dimensions, branch points, and distribution within the breast (Figs. 1-2 and 1-3). Some ducts attenuate close to the nipple, whereas others are highly arborized, draining multiple quadrants of the breast. Following major subareolar duct excision, ductal remnants can be imaged within the nipple and for variable lengths in the subareolar area (Fig. 1-4). Although our experience with ductography during pregnancy and lactation is limited, we have noted that the ducts are arborized and tortuous without significant dilation.[3,7]

Solitary, intraductal papillomas are the most common cause of spontaneous nipple discharge. Ductographically, papillomas can produce complete ductal obstruction (usually with an identifiable meniscus), filling defect(s), ductal expansion and distortion,

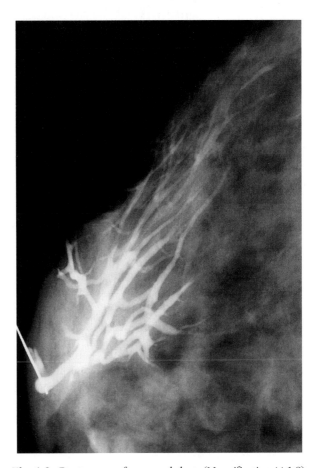

Fig. 1-2. Ductogram of a normal duct. (Magnification × 1.8)

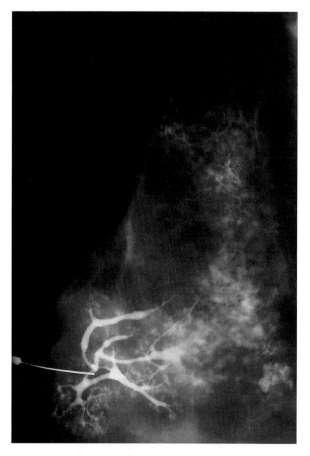

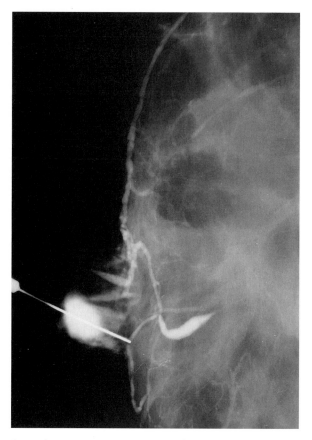

Fig. 1-3. Ductogram of a normal duct with significant parenchymal distribution and "contrast blush" (thought to reflect contrast material within normal lobules). Although infrequently seen, "lobular blushing" is thought to be a normal finding. Normal ducts are characterized by significant variation in distribution, luminal dimensions, and branch points. (Magnification × 1.8)

Fig. 1-4. Ductogram in patient after a major subareolar duct excision. Filling of ductal remnants and lymphatic channels surrounding the nipple with contrast are seen. (Magnification × 1.8)

or less commonly, duct wall irregularity[3,7] (Figs. 1-5 and 1-6). Ducts containing papillomas show variable degrees of dilation typically involving the segment of duct between the papilloma and the nipple; however, all segments of the duct can be dilated. With fibrocystic change, the second most common cause of spontaneous nipple discharge, diffuse duct wall irregularities secondary to varying degrees of epithelial hyperplasia, as well the opacification of cysts (Fig. 1-7), can be seen ductographically. Dilated ducts with a somewhat pruned appearance, tapering relatively close to the nipple, characterize duct ectasia[3,7] (Fig. 1-8). Ductographic findings of breast cancer overlap those of papillomas.

Abrupt ductal cut-off, usually with a mass at the site of the cut-off, contrast extravasation, and displacement of opacified ducts should be added to the list of findings associated with breast cancer[7,8] (Fig. 1-9).

With the newer ultrasound units, it may be reasonable to use ultrasound in the initial evaluation of patients with spontaneous nipple discharge. Intraductal lesions can be demonstrated in some patients (Fig. 1-10). Although cannulation of the duct is usually easier and painless when performed through the nipple, percutaneous cannulation of the duct can be accomplished under ultrasound guidance if discharge cannot be elicited on the day the patient presents for diagnostic evaluation or preoperative ductography. Because this percutaneous approach is usually more uncomfortable and can be painful, lido-

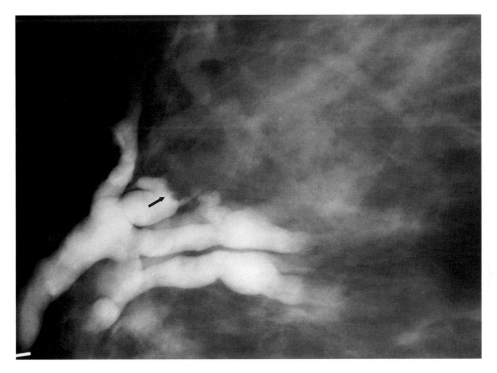

Fig. 1-5. Ductogram demonstrating a lesion (*arrow*) obstructing one of the branches of the cannulated duct. The contrast outlines the leading edge of the papilloma, creating a meniscus-like appearance. There is also diffuse duct ectasia. (Magnification × 1.8)

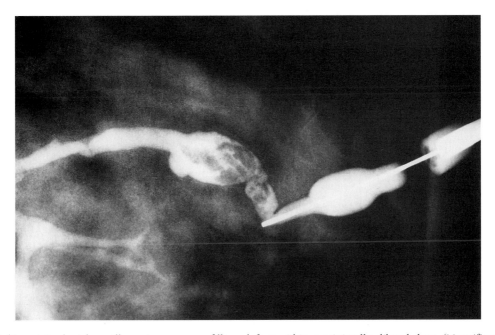

Fig. 1-6. Solitary intraductal papilloma is seen as a filling defect within a minimally dilated duct. (Magnification × 1.8)

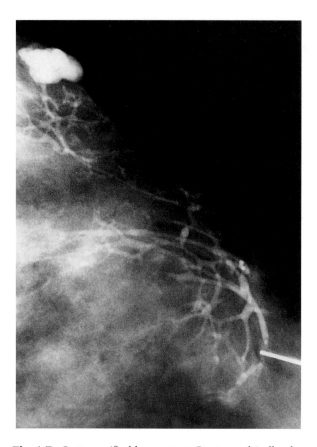

Fig. 1-7. Cyst opacified by contrast. Ductographically, the duct is otherwise normal. These patients may relate the development of a "lump" that disappears after several episodes of discharge. Presumably, the cyst is decompressing spontaneously through the nipple.

caine should be used in the skin and subareolar area, as well as combined with Conray 60 for intraductal injection (1:3 lidocaine:Conray 60).

As our experiences and observations during ductography increase, it has become clear that a considerable amount of ductal physiology has yet to be understood. One such experience is the occurrence of pseudolesions (false-positive ductograms): multiple filling defects throughout the opacified duct or a diffusely irregular (rat-bitten) duct that cannot be reproduced (Fig. 1-11) on preoperative ductography (see below). Inspissated secretions, blood clots, or muscular contractions may account for these pseudolesions; however, the exact etiology has yet to be determined.[3,7]

False-negative ductograms can result if the wrong duct is cannulated. This error can occur if the abnormal duct orifice is closely apposed to other ductal openings on the nipple surface. Correlation with the clinical presentation is critical in minimizing false-negative studies. A normal ductogram in a patient presenting with a long-standing history of significant spontaneous nipple discharge and an identifiable trigger point that elicits brisk nipple discharge may reflect cannulation of the wrong duct. Re-evaluation of these patients with ductography is appropriate, particularly if the discharge continues.[3,7]

If meticulous technique is used during cannulation, ductal perforation with contrast extravasation is rare. The patient usually experiences pain, as attempts are made to advance the cannula, and a burning sensa-

Fig. 1-8. Duct ectasia. Ductal distension involves the subareolar portion of the opacified duct. The smaller branches of the duct appear unremarkable.

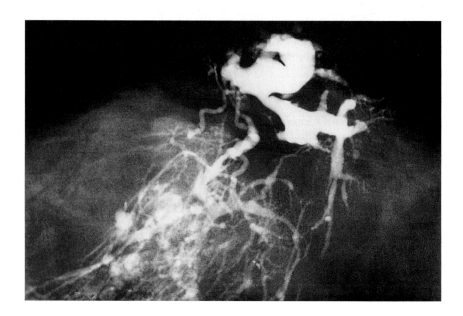

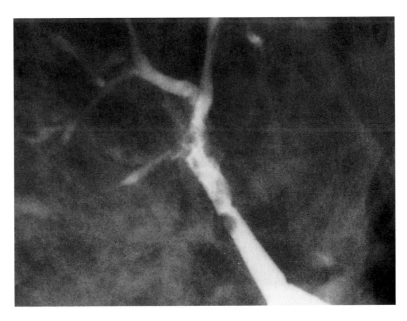

Fig. 1-9. Low-grade, ductal carcinoma in situ (cribriform pattern). Multiple filling defects and ductal wall irregularity seen ductographically in a patient with spontaneous nipple discharge and a normal mammogram.

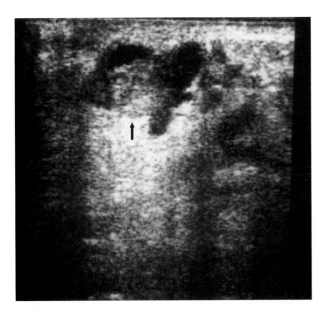

Fig. 1-10. Intraductal lesion demonstrated ultrasonographically (*arrow*). If nipple discharge cannot be reproduced percutaneously, ultrasound-guided contrast injection for diagnostic evaluation or preoperative localization can be accomplished.

can be rescheduled, or recannulation can be attempted after 15 to 20 minutes. Because only a small amount of contrast is extravasated, it is readily absorbed. Occasionally, if contrast is injected rapidly or forcefully, or if too much contrast is injected, peripheral extravasation can occur distal to an otherwise normal duct. In these patients, the cannulation is atraumatic, and the burning sensation is not present as contrast is first injected. Opacification of lymphatics and venous structures can also occur with forceful contrast injections.[3,7]

Multiple, relatively round, rather lucent filling defects, which shift in position between films (particularly if the breast is massaged), are air bubbles. If there are many air bubbles (Fig. 1-13), it is best to reschedule the patient for another examination. If only one or two air bubbles are present close to the nipple, they do not usually present a problem, as they are unlikely to obscure or simulate true lesions. The injection of too much contrast can obscure smaller lesions (Fig. 1-14). It is advisable, therefore, to inject small amounts of contrast. Additional contrast can be used as needed for adequate ductal evaluation.[3,7]

PREOPERATIVE DUCTOGRAPHY

tion as contrast is injected. A subareolar contrast blush (Fig. 1-12) is seen mammographically, usually without associated ductal opacification. The patient

Preoperative ductograms using a 1:1 methylene blue/Conray 60 are performed routinely in patients

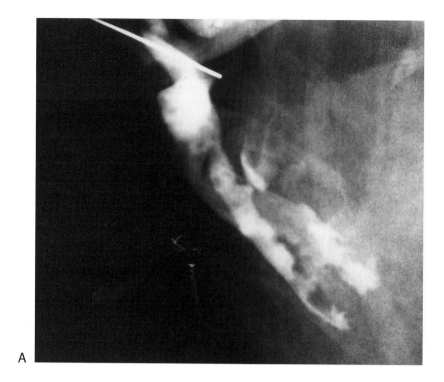

A

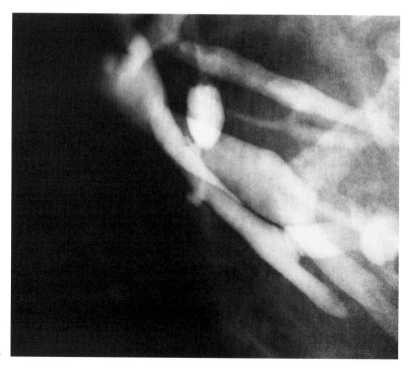

B

Fig. 1-11. (A) Diagnostic ductogram demonstrating multiple intraductal filling defects and duct wall irregularity. (Magnification × 1.8) **(B)** Diffuse ductal changes are not confirmed on recannulation of the discharging duct preoperatively. The etiology of these "pseudolesions" has yet to be established. After meticulous histologic evaluation, mild epithelial hyperplastic changes were diagnosed with no focal intraductal or intramural lesions.

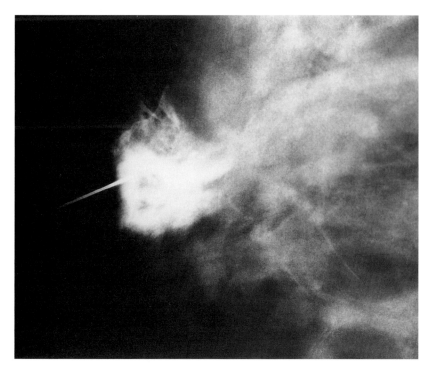

Fig. 1-12. Subareolar contrast extravasation after traumatic ductal cannulation. The patient experiences pain during the cannulation and burning when contrast is injected.

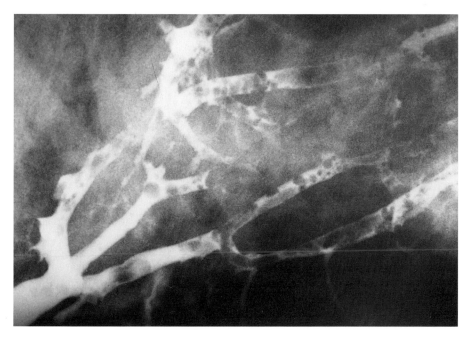

Fig. 1-13. Numerous air bubbles intraductally limit the ability to identify "true" intraductal lesions. When this occurs it is best to reschedule the patient.

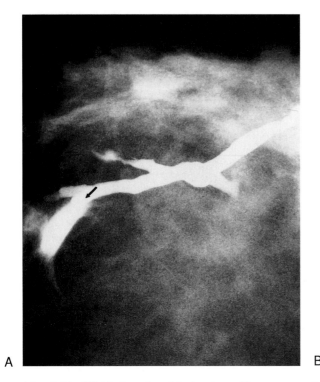
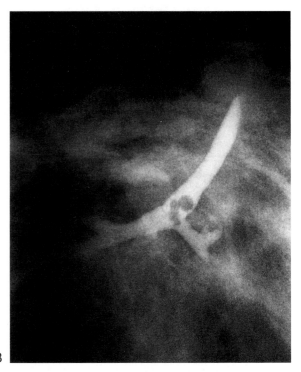

A   B

Fig. 1-14. (A) No intraductal lesion is readily apparent. Some contrast extravasation (*arrow*) is seen distal to what appears otherwise to be a normal duct. This "peripheral" extravasation suggests overinjection. (Magnification × 1.8) **(B)** Re-evaluation of the patient using a smaller amount of contrast demonstrates a filling defect confirmed preoperatively. Histologically, a papilloma was diagnosed. If too much contrast is injected at the onset of the examination, small lesions can be obscured. (Magnification × 1.8)

with suspected papillomas or breast cancer on diagnostic ductograms. The Conray 60 confirms the cannulation of the abnormal duct, and methylene blue stains the duct for the surgeon. In patients with lesions far removed from the nipple or a lesion several branch points from the main subareolar duct, the ductogram can be used to guide a preoperative wire localization (Fig. 1-15). The goal of these maneuvers is to guarantee removal of discharge-producing lesions for accurate histologic evaluation without sacrificing significant amounts of breast tissue.[3,7]

Communication among the therapeutic team members is important in managing patients with nipple discharge. The radiologist and surgeon must communicate on the ductographic findings, the appropriate preoperative localization procedure, and surgical approach to ensure complete removal of all potential intraductal lesions. Likewise, the radiologist and pathologist must communicate to guarantee adequate processing of the removed tissue. Papillomas are often small friable lesions, which can be lost easily if the specimen is not processed carefully by the pathologist. Ideally, the stained duct is dissected open by the pathologist to facilitate identification of the intraductal lesion(s).

Radiologists seem reticent to recommend ductography in patients with spontaneous nipple discharge. Ductography is a simple examination that is not associated with significant complications. It can facilitate and guide appropriate management of these patients. A little patience and persistence can have a positive impact on what is commonly a haphazard management of patients. If ductal connection with cysts or duct ectasia is documented ductographically, a biopsy may be averted. If an intraductal abnormality is identified, the number of lesions, their exact location, and their extent can be delineated and accurately localized preoperatively.

The role of ductography is undervalued by many surgeons who believe they can reliably identify abnormal ducts, intraductal lesions, and the extent of

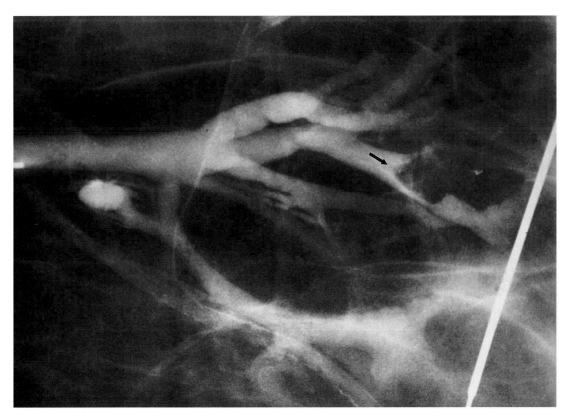

Fig. 1-15. Small intraductal lesion in a side branch of a highly arborized duct (*arrow*). Preoperative ductography with undiluted Conray 60 is used to guide a preoperative wire localization. In this patient, the reinforced segment of a modified Kopans wire is just posterior to the intraductal lesion. This maneuver ensures that the lesion of concern is excised and histologically evaluated.

these lesions in the duct through visual, intraoperative inspection of subareolar ducts. This viewpoint can be held only by those who have no conception of the variation in ductal anatomy, location, and the number of lesions seen routinely during ductography. Ducts can have a widely diverging anatomic distribution, with lesions in opposite breast quadrants 4 to 12 cm from the nipple. If our goal is accurate histologic evaluation of intraductal lesions producing discharge through precise localization and excision, ductography must be considered carefully in their preoperative evaluation.

ACKNOWLEDGMENTS

Linda Bond helped in the preparation of this manuscript.

REFERENCES

1. Cardenosa G, Eklund GW. Benign papillary neoplasms of the breast: mammographic findings. Radiology 1991; 181:751–755.
2. Leis HP, Cammarate A, LaRaja RD. Nipple discharge: significance and treatment. Breast 1985; 11:6–12.
3. Cardenosa G, Doudna C, Eklund GW. Ductography of the breast: technique and findings. Am J Roentgenol 1994; 162:1081–1087.
4. Tabar L, Dean PB, Zoltan P. Galactography: the diagnostic procedure of choice for nipple discharge. Radiology 1983; 149:31–38.
5. Haagensen CD. Diseases of the Breast, 3rd Ed. WB Saunders, Philadelphia, 1886:136–175.
6. Cardenosa G, Eklund GW. Ductography. Appl Radiol September 1992; 24–29.
7. Cardenosa G, Eklund GW. Interventional procedures in breast imaging (part II): ductography, cyst aspiration and pneumocystography and fine needle aspiration. In

Taveras JM, Ferrucci JT (eds). Radiology. JB Lippincott, Philadelphia, 1993.

8. Leborgne R. Estudio radiologico del sistema canalicular de la glandula mamaria normal y patologica. Montevideo, Uruguay, Impresora Uruguaya S. A., Juncal 1511, 1943 (author translation).

2 PNEUMCYSTOGRAPHY

Debra M. Ikeda

Mammography screening detects not only small breast cancers at an early stage, but also benign non-palpable breast abnormalities such as cysts. Occasionally, simple cysts are investigated for clinical reasons such as growing mass or other indications.[1] Masses undergoing ultrasonography that fulfill some, but not all, strict criteria for a cyst may prompt interventional procedures such as pneumocystography for definitive diagnosis. During pneumocystography, a needle is inserted into a breast cyst, fluid is drained, and air is injected into the cyst cavity. Mammograms of the air-filled cyst cavity, called pneumocystograms, can provide clues as to whether an intracystic mass exists, and the air injected into the cyst cavity is therapeutic.[2,3] This chapter reviews both palpable and imaging-guided cyst aspiration, including indications for their use, techniques of aspiration, possible complications, pneumocystogram interpretation, and use in patient management.

INDICATIONS FOR CYST PUNCTURE

Breast cysts are a common benign entity, occurring in 7 to 10 percent of all adult women.[4] A breast cyst is characterized by a terminal ductal lobular unit that is undergoing apocrine metaplastic changes, which results in an apocrine-lined microcyst.[4] This microcyst can grow into an enlarged fluid-filled dilated structure (cyst), which can range in size from millimeters to centimeters. On mammography, a breast cyst is an oval or round breast mass with well-circumscribed borders. On ultrasound, strict ultrasonographic criteria for a simple breast cyst include an anechoic oval or round mass with imperceptible walls and enhanced transmission of sound.[5] Simple cysts do not need further work-up or follow-up if the patient is asymptomatic.

A breast cyst is not cancerous, and breast cancer within a cyst is extremely rare.[6] A simple breast cyst is important only in that it may mimic breast cancer on screening mammography by enlarging on sequential studies, by appearing as a new mass between mammographic screenings, or by having borders that are ill-defined or obscured by adjacent glandular tissue. Such breast masses, which subsequently do not fulfill all strict ultrasonographic criteria for a breast cyst, may require further work-up by needle aspiration to confirm or exclude the presence of a simple cyst, rather than a solid lesion. Thus, careful lesion selection for breast masses undergoing aspiration and pneumocystography is important to maximize benefit from the procedure while holding down costs.

Pneumocystography can be used to evaluate cystic lesions containing internal debris, mural nodules, solid components, or lesions that have irregular walls on ultrasound. Such masses can represent complex cysts or cystic masses. Because cytologic evaluation of the cyst fluid is untrustworthy even in cysts containing intracystic carcinomas, the pneumocystogram can provide a definitive diagnosis. Any cystic masses containing solid mural components should be surgically excised; however, the decision for pneumocystography should be based on whether the procedure will affect patient management.

Pneumocystography is useful in managing symptomatic cysts that are palpable or associated with breast pain. Air injected into the cyst cavity is both diagnostic and therapeutic; more than 90 percent of such cysts do not recur after a successful pneumocystogram.[2,3] Palpable masses are often managed by the referring physician or health care professional in the office; therefore, palpable cyst aspiration in the breast-imaging suite is less common than imaging-guided aspiration.

EQUIPMENT AND PATIENT PREPARATION

Cyst aspiration requires alcohol to cleanse the skin, a 20- or 22-gauge needle long enough to reach the cyst, two syringes (one to aspirate the cyst fluid and one to inject air), gauze to hold compression on the puncture site, and a bandage. Some physicians also use extension tubing to connect the needle to the aspirating syringe, and some use a syringe holder for easier aspiration. Lidocaine (1 percent) or other local anesthetic can be used to help decrease the sting of the initial needle insertion.

Patient preparation also consists of prior clinical breast examination by the referring physician or health care professional, because aspiration results in hemorrhage, which may produce bruising and a mass. These masses can result in confusing clinical findings if the patient is examined for the first time after aspiration. Because the breast is usually repalpated a month or more after aspiration by the referring physician to exclude cyst recurrence, an initial baseline breast physical examination is crucial. Aspiration is contraindicated in patients who cannot remain motionless for the procedure, or when the lesion is sufficiently deep or close to the chest wall so that aspiration cannot be accomplished safely. In general, the procedure is contraindicated in patients on anticoagulant therapy.

PALPABLE CYST ASPIRATION TECHNIQUE

This technique has been implemented successfully for many years in clinical practice. With the patient lying supine, the physician palpates the breast cyst to be aspirated and cleans the overlying skin with alcohol. The cyst is held firmly in one hand, while the other hand inserts a needle into the mass (Fig. 2-1). Care must be taken to ensure that the mass is far enough away from the chest wall to prevent pneumothorax. If the mass is near the chest wall, it can be gripped firm-

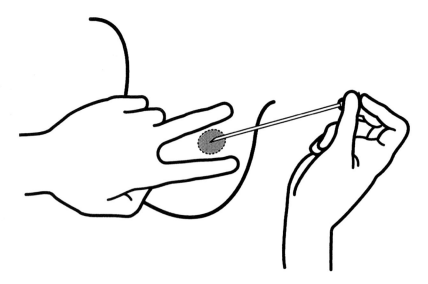

Fig. 2–1. Diagrammatic representation of a palpable cyst aspiration. The mass is held firmly between two fingers of one hand while the other hand inserts the needle until fluid wells up in the needle hub. After fluid is aspirated, air can be injected into the cyst cavity.

ly between the thumb and forefinger, holding it away from the thorax during puncture, or the patient can be repositioned so that the mass falls away from the chest wall in a dependent fashion. Alternatively, the needle may be inserted into the mass parallel, rather than perpendicular, to the chest wall.

As soon as cyst fluid wells up in the needle hub, a syringe or extension tubing and syringe are attached to the needle. The needle is held firmly, to prevent forward motion as the syringe is attached. The syringe plunger is withdrawn, aspirating the fluid until the cyst cavity is emptied completely. The syringe is detached carefully, while the other hand holds the needle in place to prevent the needle tip from moving out of the empty cyst cavity. The amount of cyst fluid in the syringe is measured and placed into a tube, and a second syringe is filled with a slightly lesser amount of air. The air is then injected through the indwelling needle into the cyst cavity. The needle is withdrawn from the cyst without detaching the now-empty syringe, and light pressure is held on the puncture site to prevent bleeding.

Craniocaudal and mediolateral pneumocystograms taken after cyst aspiration show an air-filled, smooth-walled cavity without intracystic masses. Bubbles may form in the cyst cavity during air injection if there is residual fluid in the cavity (Fig. 2-2). If the cyst fluid is clear and nonbloody, and there are no intracystic masses on the pneumocystogram, the cyst fluid can be discarded, because studies have shown that cytologic analysis of such fluid is almost invariably acellular.[3] The fluid should be sent for cytologic analysis if there are intracystic masses, if the cyst fluid is bloody or turbid, or if there are clinical indications to do so.

Repalpation of the air-filled cyst ensures that the mass prompting aspiration has resolved. An air-filled cyst is not palpable because unlike fluid, the air cannot distend the cyst cavity to produce a mass. Thus, if a palpable mass remains after cyst aspiration, either residual fluid remains in the cyst or a cyst next to a palpable solid mass has been punctured.[7] Reaspiration ensures that all palpable findings have been evaluated. If the palpable finding proves to be solid, further investigation with mammography, ultrasound, or biopsy is necessary.

GRID-COORDINATE ASPIRATION OF CYSTS

Commonly used for needle/hook-wire preoperative localization of nonpalpable breast lesions, the grid-

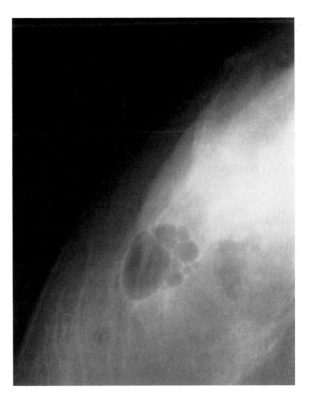

Fig. 2-2. Pneumocystogram of a multichambered, smooth-walled cyst containing bubbles caused by air injection into residual cyst fluid. Note the lobulated cyst wall borders.

coordinate technique uses a fenestrated compression plate with an alpha-numeric grid placed along the sides of an open fenestration or aperture. First, the craniocaudal and lateral views are reviewed to estimate the shortest distance from the lesion to the skin, and the projection in which the lesion will be punctured is chosen. The aperture of the grid-coordinate plate is placed on the skin closest to the lesion to allow the needle to traverse the shortest distance to the mass. Tight compression holds the breast in place without causing patient discomfort. Black marks in indelible ink are made around the opening of the aperture on the patient's skin to verify that patient position does not change during the procedure.

A film in this projection shows whether or not the lesion is located within the aperture of the coordinate plate. If the lesion is not within the aperture, the technologist repositions the breast. Once the lesion is in the aperture, the location of the lesion is calculated on the film by looking at the grid coordinates. A line is drawn through the lesion to the edges of the coordinates on the film (Fig. 2-3). The coordinates are then located on the patient's skin, and a small mark on the

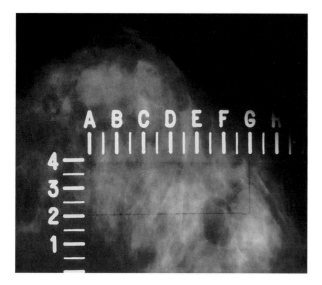

Fig. 2-3. Alpha-numeric grid localization method for cyst aspiration. The cyst lies in the grid-localization plate aperture at coordinates 2.0, G.0. Note the normal pneumocystogram of a cyst previously punctured at coordinates 2.0, F.0.

skin is made with indelible black ink. The skin is then wiped with iodine or alcohol. A small amount of 1 percent lidocaine (2 to 3 cc) is mixed with 0.3 cc of 8.4901 bicarbonate solution to help minimize the sting the patient feels on initial injection of local anesthetic. A skin wheal is raised by injection of the lidocaine and bicarbonate mixture at the indelible ink mark, which will be the location of the needle entry point.

The 90-degree orthogonal view determines the lesion depth. The location of the lesion is estimated as lying in the upper third, the middle third, or lower third of the breast near the chosen needle entry point. By measuring the thickness of the patient's breast between the image receptor and the rise of the skin above the plate aperture with a ruler, the breast thickness in compression can be determined. Using this number, the depth of the lesion can be estimated; for example, if the breast is 6 cm thick in compression and the lesion is in the middle third of the breast, then the lesion must lie within the first 3 cm deep to the skin (Fig. 2-4). Using this depth estimation plus 1 cm additional length, a needle is selected to reach the lesion. Thus, for our hypothetical lesion, the needle would be 4 cm long.

Using the positioning light, the hub of the needle is placed over the needle shaft so that its shadow projects over the shaft. This maneuver ensures that

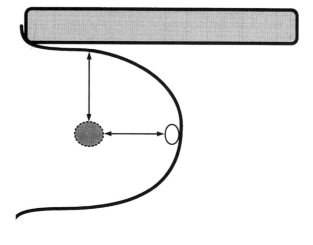

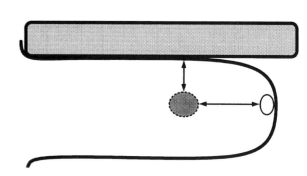

Fig. 2-4. Estimating cyst depth during breast compression. The upper figure shows the cyst in the middle of the breast on a standard mediolateral view. With compression, the distance from the skin to the mass decreases, but the mass remains in the middle of the compressed breast. Thus, needle depth required to penetrate the mass is calculated from the thickness of the breast in compression. If the thickness of the breast in compression is 6 cm, the mass will be about 3 cm from the skin surface.

the needle will be straight while inserted. The needle is inserted to the correct depth or until fluid wells up through the hub. If no fluid is obtained, the needle is inserted 1 cm deep to the initial estimated lesion depth. If fluid wells up through the needle hub, a syringe is attached and the fluid is aspirated and measured. A second syringe injects a slightly lesser volume of air and the needle is withdrawn. Pneumocystogram films confirm that all of the fluid has been drained.

If fluid is not obtained when the needle is passed initially into the lesion, a repeat film can be obtained to ensure that the needle tip projects over the lesion. If the tip is not within the lesion, the needle is repositioned. If the tip projects over the lesion and there is no fluid, a larger gauge needle can be used to aspirate tenacious, thick fluid. If fluid is not obtained with a larger gauge, properly positioned needle, the lesion is assumed to be solid and is managed appropriately. Alternatively, ultrasound can be used to scan through the compression plate aperture to confirm the lesion location and determine lesion depth (Fig. 2-5).

With the breast in compression, the cyst is flattened and the fluid within it placed under some tension. The fluid may empty quickly on needle penetration, and the needle tip can move out of the cavity as it decreases in size (Fig. 2-6). To avoid this possibility, the needle should be held carefully with one hand as the syringe is attached or when the needle is manipulated.

Pneumocystography films are essential to confirm that the cyst has been completely drained and to evaluate the cyst lining. Air outside the cavity is also

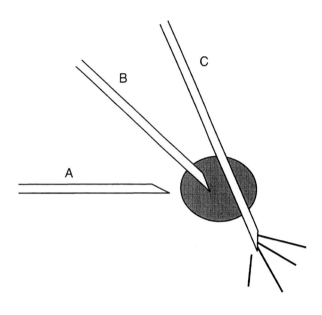

Fig. 2-6. Diagrammatic demonstration of failure to aspirate fluid by **(A)** no penetration of the mass by the needle and **(C)** passage of the needle through the mass. In some cases, after correct needle placement **(B),** the needle tip can move out of the cyst wall cavity as in **(A),** and **(C).** The air introduced for pneumocystography will be outside of the mass, dissecting into the soft tissues of the breast.

visible on the pneumocystogram and has the appearance of subcutaneous emphysema, but will resolve within a few days and causes no known harm to the patient (Fig. 2-7).

STEREOTAXIC FINE-NEEDLE ASPIRATION

Similar to core biopsy, fine-needle aspiration of breast cysts can be performed with a stereotaxic device. These devices calculate the three-dimensional location of the cyst from images obtained at 15 degrees off the perpendicular. The patient may be either upright or prone in these devices. After location of the cyst is calculated, the skin is prepared and lidocaine is injected into the skin. A fine-needle is inserted into the target lesion with a 22-gauge, 3.5-in (9 cm) spinal needle. Repeat stereo films are obtained to

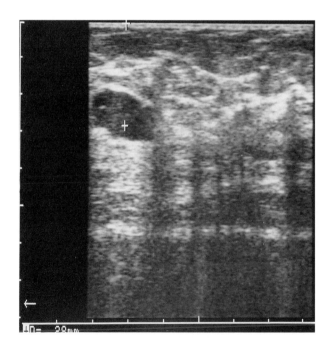

Fig. 2-5. Ultrasound image obtained through the aperture of a grid-coordinate plate can verify mass location and depth from the skin. In this case, the ultrasound image taken through the grid-localization aperture at the coordinates 2.0, G.0 in Figure 2-3 shows a hypoechoic mass, which lies 28 mm deep to the skin. This technique allows the operator to select a needle long enough to reach the mass.

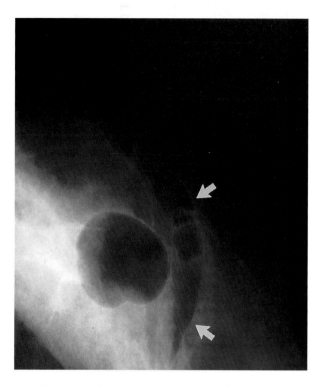

Fig. 2-7. Magnified pneumocystogram of a large simple cyst. Adjacent to the cyst is extravasated air in the soft tissues of the breast (*arrows*). The air will be resorbed by the body in a few days.

confirm that the needle tip is within the lesion (Fig. 2-8). If positioning is incorrect, the needle position is adjusted. The needle is inserted slowly until fluid wells up through the hub. Occasionally, because of flattening of the cyst in compression, the initial needle insertion may not penetrate the lesion. If this happens, the tip can be advanced 5 to 10 mm deeper than the initially calculated location of the lesion. Once this fluid wells up through the needle hub, the cyst should be aspirated in the usual manner. Air can be injected through the needle while it is still in the stereotaxic device. The needle is withdrawn and pneumocystogram films are obtained (Fig. 2-9).

CYST ASPIRATION UNDER ULTRASOUND GUIDANCE

Preparation of the patient for ultrasound-guided aspiration is similar to other methods, except that the patient is placed supine with her hand behind her head, and the lesion must be placed so that there is no possibility of traversing the chest wall with the aspirating needle. In addition, the ultrasound transducer must be sterilized with iodine or other solution, or covered with a sterile, commercially available plastic or latex sleeve in which ultrasound gel has been

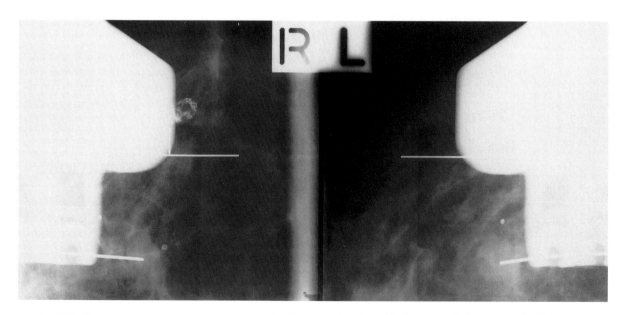

Fig. 2-8. Stereotactic cyst aspiration. Stereotactic views (both taken 15 degrees off the perpendicular) verify that the needle lies within the cyst. If fluid is not obtained, the Z axis is advanced deeper to enter the compressed cyst. If fluid is still not obtained, core biopsy of a solid lesion can be performed.

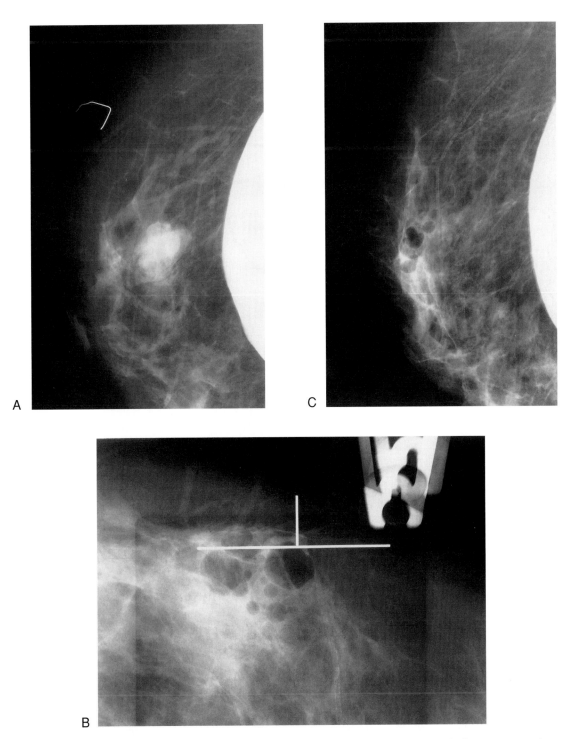

Fig. 2-9. (A) Smoothly lobulated moderately dense mass in the mid portion of the right breast near a silicone implant. The stereotactically guided aspiration can be performed safely if the cyst can be compressed away from the implant edge. **(B)** Craniocaudal view of the same breast in Figure A in the stereotactic compression plate. Following aspiration of fluid and injection of air, this view shows multiple, smooth-walled, air-containing cyst cavities. **(C)** Final right mediolateral oblique pneumocystogram film shows a normal pneumocystogram. The intact silicone implant is well away from the region of the procedure.

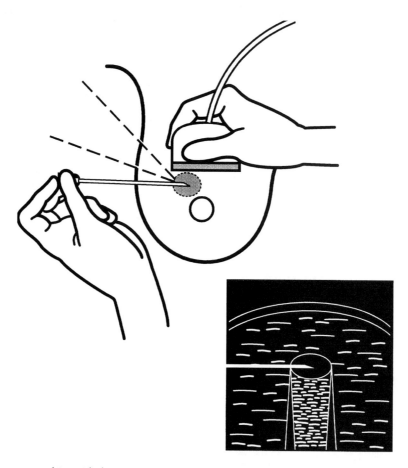

Fig. 2-10. Ultrasonographic-guided mass aspiration technique. Performed with one or two operators, the hand holding the ultrasound transducer should remain stable while needle insertion takes place. The needle should be parallel to and in the middle of the axis of the transducer to allow optimal needle visualization. Under real-time ultrasound guidance, the fluid can be aspirated. The mass will disappear, and air injected for pneumocystography will create a pattern of distal acoustic shadowing.

inserted. Other manufacturers suggest that the transducer be covered with plastic wrap and sterilized with iodine. Liberal iodine solution or sterile saline on the skin can be used as the coupling material for the sterile transducer during scanning.

After sterilization, the lesion is placed in the middle of the scan field. The skin next to the transducer is sterilized, and a needle is passed into the lesion under direct ultrasound guidance. To visualize the shaft of the needle, one hand or operator holds the transducer steady, and the second hand passes the needle so that the shaft travels along the long axis of the transducer. The needle shaft should be placed in the middle of the short axis transducer to ensure its visualization (Fig. 2-10). If the shaft of the needle cannot be seen, the

transducer can be rotated to find the shaft of the needle, and the needle can be repositioned. Once the needle has traversed the cyst wall (Fig. 2-11A), a technologist attaches either a syringe or tubing to aspirate the fluid. After aspiration, air is injected into the cyst using a second syringe, producing a complex echogenic pattern of distal acoustic shadowing (Fig. 2-11B). After the needle is removed and pressure applied, pneumocystograms can be obtained.

INTERPRETATION

Pneumocystograms should be obtained in both craniocaudal and lateral projections, showing an air-filled

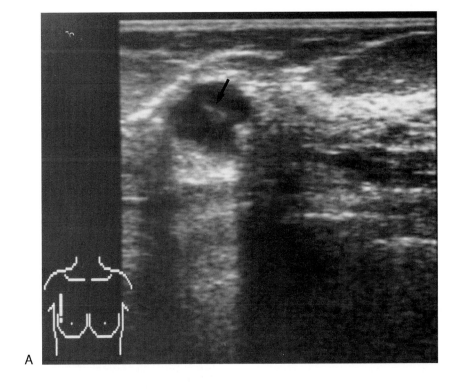

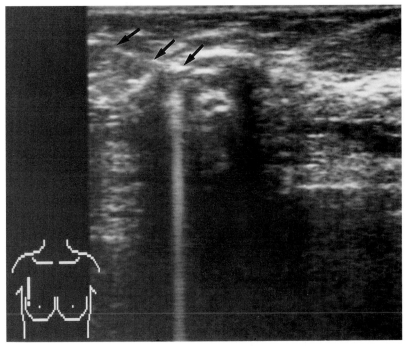

Fig. 2-11. (A) Ultrasonographically guided aspiration of a hypoechoic mass. The needle tip (*arrow*) lies within the mass. **(B)** Ultrasonographic image after aspiration of fluid and injection of air into the cyst shown in Fig. A. In the region of the hypoechoic mass is a complex echogenic pattern of distal acoustic shadowing, which has the appearance of the air injected into the aspirated cavity. The needle through which air was injected is still present (*arrows*).

cavity with imperceptible walls and no intracystic masses. Occasionally, the fluid is not completely aspirated and an air-fluid level results. Reaspiration will allow evaluation of the cyst walls. The pneumocystogram ensures that all walls of the cyst are clear, that there are no intracystic masses, that the location of the aspirated lesion corresponds to the lesion originally prompting biopsy, and that the correct lesion has been punctured and proven to be a cyst. In these cases, the woman can be returned to routine mammographic screening.

The pneumocystogram films and the fluid appearance should be correlated with the clinical history and the mammographic impression. If the cyst displays suspicious mammographic or clinical features, cytologic examination should be obtained and correlated. Cytologic examination should always be obtained if the fluid is bloody. If the pneumocystogram and cytology from the bloody fluids are normal, and the clinical features of the patient are not suspicious, the patient is seen at 6 months for a unilateral mammogram to evaluate for cyst recurrence. Recurrent cysts are reaspirated and cytology repeated. If the results are still normal, the mammograms are again repeated at 6 months. A third cyst recurrence prompts surgical excision, particularly if the cyst fluid has been bloody.

If the lesion contains an intracystic mass, cytologic examination may not be definitive[3] (Fig. 2-12). Thus, all intracystic masses require needle localization and surgical biopsy for histologic diagnosis, even if cytologic results are benign.

CONCLUSION

Fine-needle aspiration of breast cysts is fast and definitive when performed correctly. Essential steps in cyst aspiration include cyst puncture, complete aspiration of the fluid, and inflation with air. The postaspiration pneumocystogram films confirm that the lesion in question was punctured and that the cyst contains no intracystic masses. In clinical practice, these procedures can be definitive for women, who can be returned to routine screening after cyst puncture.

ACKNOWLEDGMENT

Robyn L. Birdwell, M.D., assisted in the preparation of this manuscript.

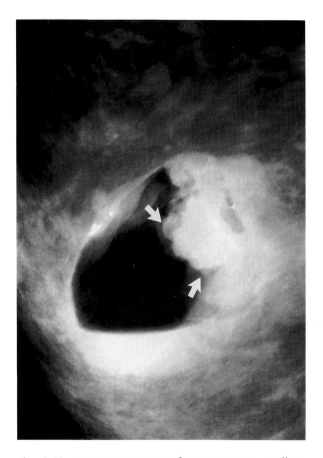

Fig. 2-12. Pneumocystogram of an intracystic papilloma (*arrows*) within an incompletely aspirated cavity containing an air-fluid level. Note the multilobulated mass extending from the cyst wall into the air-filled cyst cavity. Cytologic examination of the aspirated blood-tinged fluid showed nonspecific benign cells, demonstrating the importance of the pneumocystogram for diagnosis.

REFERENCES

1. Fajardo L, Jackson V, Hunter T. Interventional procedures in diseases of the breast: needle biopsy, pneumocystography, and galactography. Am J Roentgenol 1992; 158:1231–1238.
2. Ikeda D, Helvie M, Adler D, et al. The role of fine-needle aspiration and pneumocystography in the treatment of impalpable breast cysts. Am J Roentgenol 1992; 158:1239–1241.
3. Tabar L, Pentek Z, Dean P. The diagnostic and therapeutic values of breast cyst puncture and pneumocystography. Radiology 1981; 141:659–663.

4. Hess J, Sedghinasab M, Moe R, et al. Growth factor profiles in breast cyst fluid identify women with increased breast cancer risk. Am J Surg 1994; 167:523–530.

5. Meyer J, Christian R, Frenna T, et al. Image-guided aspiration of solitary occult breast 'cysts.' Arch Surg 1992; 127:433–435.

6. Sterns E. The natural history of macroscopic cysts in the breast. Surg Gynecol Obstet 1992; 174:36–40.

7. Angeid-Backman E, Ikeda D, Andersson I, Linell F. Complementary roles of mammography and physical examination in palpable cyst aspirations. Breast Dis 1992; 5:1–9.

3 NEEDLE LOCALIZATION FOR BREAST BIOPSY

D. David Dershaw

The utilization of screening mammography has led to the detection of nonpalpable abnormalities that require biopsy. Much of this book is devoted to techniques by which the radiologist can perform tissue sampling of these lesions to determine whether they require surgical intervention. In many facilities, however, these procedures may not be available. Moreover, for some patients, surgical biopsy may be more appropriate than percutaneous tissue sampling. In these situations preoperative needle location is indicated.

The goal of preoperative needle localization is twofold. First, the procedure is designed to direct the surgeon to the appropriate site within the breast so that the suspicious lesion is removed successfully. Second, because most of these abnormalities are benign or, if malignant, may be treated with breast-conserving techniques, needle localization enables the abnormality to be removed while excising a minimal volume of tissue, thereby minimizing postsurgical deformity.

Multiple steps should be carried out to ensure a successful needle localization with minimal patient discomfort and anxiety. The radiologist performing this procedure needs to routinely examine mammograms before patients are accepted for the procedure to be certain that a complete imaging work-up has been completed and that the scheduled biopsy is indicated. Both the radiologist and surgeon should agree on and be comfortable with the localization technique to ensure that an accurate localization is performed. Specimen radiography is an essential part of the excision of many lesions and must be performed during the surgical procedure. A decision about the appropriateness of performing a frozen section analysis of the specimen should be made, often in consultation with the pathologist.

PRELOCALIZATION ANALYSIS OF THE PATIENT

Before the patient arrives for the localization procedure, the films on which a biopsy has been recommended must be reviewed to determine that the procedure is indicated and that the lesion can be seen on two orthogonal views so that it can be located in the breast. In addition, the appropriate approach needs to be determined before the procedure begins. If films are inadequate to determine the site of the lesion within the breast, additional images should be obtained. The policy in our department is to fully work up patients before they arrive for needle localization and not delay final assessment until the time of localization. The importance of this review is reinforced by one series of 603 patients referred for needle localization.[1] Among these women, biopsy was cancelled in 9 percent because a lesion was not present, the lesion was in the skin, or it was a cyst and could be aspirated. Review of studies before the day of the procedure diminishes patient anxiety about whether or not a biopsy is necessary and allows inappropriate procedures to be cancelled, resulting in more efficient utilization of surgical and radiographic facilities.

According to published series, the rate of discovery of carcinoma (positive predictive value) on needle localized biopsy should range from about 20 to 30 percent of women undergoing the procedure. These data actually reflect the positive predictive value of a biopsy recommendation. Multiple factors influence this percentage, but it must be established for each practice. If fewer than 20 percent of women undergoing needle localized biopsy have cancer, lesions that may be better suited to short-term mammographic follow-up or lesions that are obviously benign are being sent to biopsy. If large numbers of women undergoing needle localization have cancer, indeterminate lesions are not being biopsied in sufficient numbers. In addition, the utilization of percutaneous needle biopsy techniques will result in fewer women with benign lesions undergoing needle localization; these techniques will increase the likelihood of finding cancer during needle localization.

SELECTION OF LOCALIZATION TECHNIQUE

Several techniques are available to perform needle localization. All involve positioning a needle at or close to the lesion in question and then leaving a marker in place when the needle is removed. The procedure is usually performed with either wire positioning or dye injection.

Wire Localization Techniques

In this technique a wire encased in a needle is positioned in the breast. After appropriate positioning, the needle is withdrawn, and the wire is left in place. A length of wire extends beyond the skin and is secured in place. At surgery the lesion can be reached by dissection along the wire or by a periareolar approach. Multiple wires can be placed in the breast to mark the margins of large lesions (e.g., suspicious microcalcifications) that are being excised. The wire positioning remains secure in most patients, but some migration of the wire may occur, especially in large, fatty breasts where anchoring of the hook may not be as secure as in more glandular or fibrous breasts.

Complications with wire localization are rare. If a long length of wire is not left beyond the skin surface, the wire may retract into the breast, requiring repeat localization to find the original wire. Migration of wires that have retracted into the breast may occur, and these wires may migrate outside the breast.[2] Penetration of a wire into the pleural space also has been reported.[3] More commonly, the wire can be transected during surgery, with the deep portion retracting into the breast and becoming lost.[4]

Dye Localization Techniques

Dye localization is performed by injecting 0.1 to 0.2 ml of dye and radiographic contrast through a needle positioned at the site of the lesion. The injected solution consists of 50 to 60 percent iodinated contrast material and 40 to 50 percent blue dye. The contrast material is visible on the postlocalization mammogram, and the dye is visible during the biopsy. Dyes that have been used in this technique include methylene blue, toluidine blue, Evans blue, and isocyanide green. Methylene blue may interfere with estrogen-receptor, protein-binding capacity assay.[5] Evans blue and toluidine blue have been criticized because they may diffuse too rapidly.

The most important criticism of this technique is that dye may diffuse within the breast, making localization less precise. Complications specific to dye injection have not been reported. Allergic reactions during the procedure, either to the dye or to the contrast material, have not been reported. If patients refuse iodinated contrast, a small volume of air can be mixed with the dye, which will be visible on the mammogram after the localization.

PERFORMING THE LOCALIZATION

The woman undergoing breast needle localization needs to be awake and cooperative. Preoperative sedation should not be given before the localization. The procedure should be explained to her, and informed consent should be obtained. Local anesthetic may be used, but one study reported that patients thought the procedure was more painful when a subcutaneous injection of local anesthetic was given than when it was not.[6] The localization procedure and biopsy should be performed on the same day. Localizations using the dye technique should be performed within a few hours of surgery because the dye may diffuse or resorb. The patient should be in a sitting position. The decision regarding positioning of the needle can be made independent of the surgical approach. The site at which the needle is inserted should be chosen to try to minimize the skin-to-lesion distance. Because the nipple and areola are the most painful areas through which to insert a needle, they should be avoided, if possible.

It is often useful to obtain a 90-degree lateral view to help estimate the depth of the lesion from the skin. The lesion depth will be demonstrated accurately on this view only for those lesions that are in the 12 and 6 o'clock axes. For other lesions, the skin-to-lesion distance will be less.

When the needle approach to the lesion has been chosen, a scout film of the breast with an alpha-numeric, fenestrated compression paddle is obtained to localize the exact site on the skin overlying the abnormality (Fig. 3-1). The patient is kept in compression while this film is developed (Fig. 3-2). Using this image, the exact site on the skin at which the needle will be introduced is marked, and the skin is cleansed with an alcohol swab.

The physician and technologist must be gloved to protect themselves and the patient during this invasive procedure. Examining gloves or sterile gloves can be used. The needle or needle/wire combination are introduced to the estimated depth of the lesion. The needle should be inserted parallel to the chest to avoid the possibility of penetrating the chest, causing pneumothorax or other complications. The needle also should be introduced so that it does not cast a shadow when illuminated by the field light on the mammography unit. The angle at which the beams of light diverge approximates the angle at which the x-rays diverge. Because only a lesion in the center of the field has been imaged with x-rays passing perpendicular to the floor, some angulation of needle is necessary to follow the course of the x-rays, especially for sites deep within the breast.

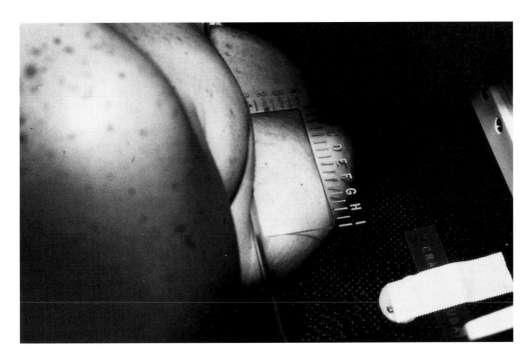

Fig. 3-1. A patient with a suspicious nodule in the lateral aspect of her breast is positioned in compression with an alpha-numeric fenestrated grid to localize the lesion in a single projection. In this case she is positioned in the craniocaudal position. A film is taken and the needle is positioned at the appropriate site in the breast. The patient will be kept in this position until a needle has been inserted and a second film taken to confirm its position.

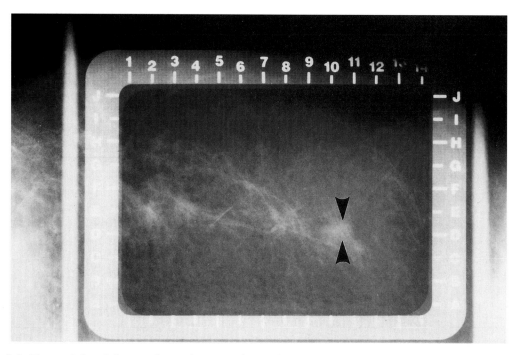

Fig. 3-2. Figures 3-3 to 3-5 were obtained as part of a needle localization of a woman with an ill-defined nodule in the upper outer quadrant of her breast. The initial film, shown here, was taken in the craniocaudal projection with an alpha-numeric compression grid. It localizes the nodule (*arrowheads*) to the D/10 coordinates.

After the needle has been positioned, two views at right angles are obtained to check the position of the needle within the breast (Fig. 3-3). If the needle cannot be introduced to the required depth while the patient is in position for the initial film, the needle should be introduced to its required depth before the second view is obtained. The patient is kept in mammographic compression and positioned for the second view, during which these images are developed. The needle tip should be positioned at least within 1 cm of the lesion (Fig. 3-4B). If the needle has been accurately placed, the wire may be introduced or the dye injected, and the needle can be withdrawn. If needle positioning is not accurate, appropriate adjustments can be made (Fig. 3-4C). Dye is introduced into the breast by attaching a TB syringe to the needle and injecting the appropriate volume of dye and contrast. For wire localization, the wire is held firmly in place while the needle is withdrawn from the breast. As the needle is withdrawn and the wire tip becomes exposed, the wire hook opens and becomes anchored in breast tissue.

If a dye localization is performed, it is common for the patient to experience stinging at the time of the of the injection. If a wire localization is performed, several centimeters of wire should be left outside the skin and should be secured to the skin surface to avoid retraction of the wire into the breast. The wire should be taped to the breast, and a piece of gauze can be used to cover the site.

After the localization has been performed, a two-view mammogram is obtained (Fig. 3-5). It is often worthwhile to perform the lateral as a 90-degree lateral rather than a mediolateral oblique because this approach gives the surgeon a more accurate impression of the location of the lesion within the breast. These films should be labeled, indicating the lesion, localizing wire or dye, and indicating the patient's position on each film. The films are sent to surgery with the patient.

If large, nonpalpable lesions or multiple lesions are being localized, multiple wires can be used to mark the margins of the lesion or lesions in the breast that need to be excised (Fig. 3-6A). The two or more

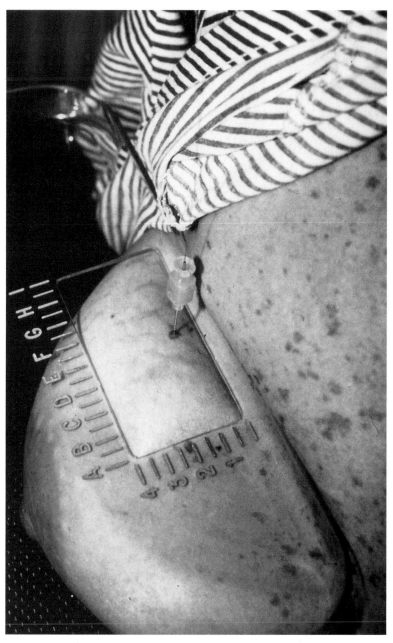

A

Fig. 3-3. (A) After a needle is positioned within the breast, a second film is taken to confirm appropriate positioning. When the compression paddle is lifted, care must be taken to avoid disturbing the position of the needle. *(Figure continues.)*

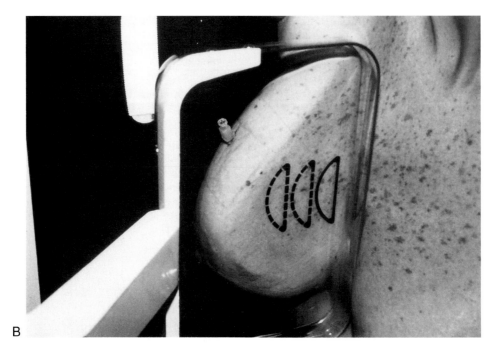

Fig. 3-3. *(Continued).* **(B)** The patient is then positioned in the orthogonal position, in this case a 90-degree lateral. The needle depth should be adjusted to what is believed to be the appropriate depth, and a film is taken to check on the needle position in this projection.

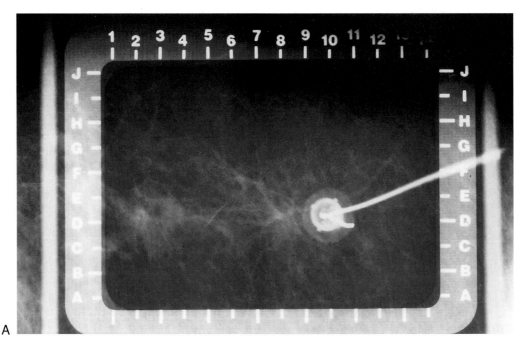

Fig. 3-4. (A) After the needle and wire have been positioned, films are taken to verify accurate positioning. Note that the needle hub actually obscures the lesion in this image. The hub is also superimposed on the needle, and only the portion of the wire outside the breast is seen in the mammogram. *(Figure continues.)*

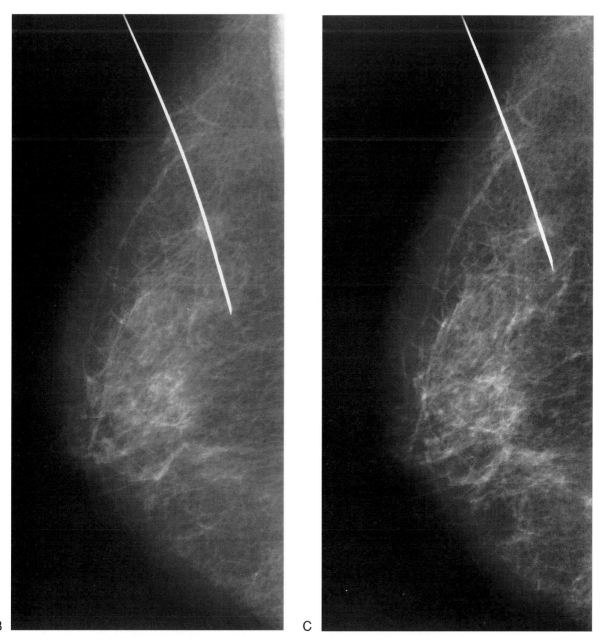

B   C

Fig. 3-4. *(Continued).* **(B)** An orthogonal mammogram, performed as a 90-degree mediolateral, demonstrates that the needle tip is deep to the suspicious lesion. **(C)** The needle has been withdrawn partially, and its tip is now in proximity to the suspicious lesion. The needle can now be withdrawn, engaging the hook wire.

wires can be placed in the breast simultaneously or serially. Multiple dye injections may not be useful, as the dye can diffuse and color a large volume of breast tissue, thereby reducing the ability to localize lesions within the breast.

SURGICAL REMOVAL OF A LOCALIZED LESION

Excision of a needle-localized lesion is usually performed as a same-day admission, obviating the need

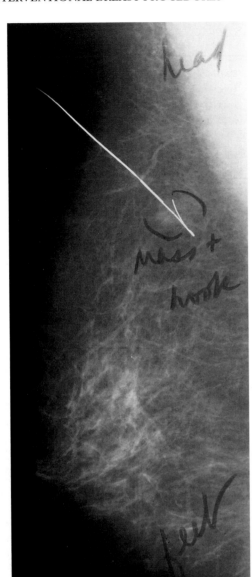
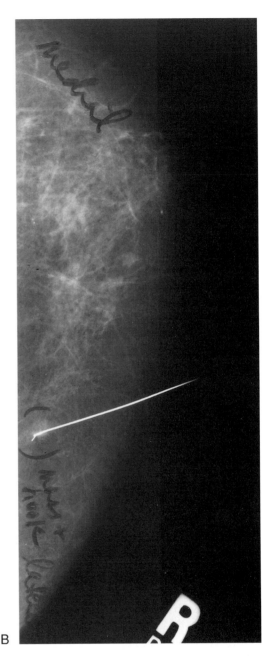

A   B

Fig. 3-5. (A) Ninety-degree mediolateral and **(B)** craniocaudal views of the breast after the wire has been positioned. The location of the wire and lesion and the positioning of the breast are labeled on these images, which are sent to surgery with the patient.

for an overnight hospital stay. Either local anesthesia, often supplemented with intravenous sedation, or general anesthesia can be used. Lesions that are very posterior in the breast may require general anesthesia.

The surgeon may cut along the length of the wire, but if the wire passes through a long distance, it may be best to avoid this approach. Care must be taken not to transect the wire. A periareolar approach is appropriate for lesions near the nipple. The volume of tissue removed should be minimal, thus avoiding deformity of the breast after surgery. When the specimen is removed, it should be marked with sutures to indicate orientation of the tissue. If malignancy is found, this technique allows assessment of contamination of margins within the tumor and facilitates re-excision. The patient should not be removed from the operating table until specimen radiography has confirmed excision of the lesion, especially when calcifications are being biopsied.

PATHOLOGIC ANALYSIS OF A LOCALIZED LESION

Following excision, removal of the lesion is confirmed with specimen radiography (Fig. 3-6B). This procedure is routine for lesions that contain calcifications. When masses are localized, examination of the specimen may reveal the mass, and specimen radiography, often requiring compression, also can be used. In malignant lesions, two orthogonal views of the specimen should be obtained to assess whether the tumor extends to the margin of resection. The pathologist also should ink the margins of the specimen to help assess whether tumor extends to the margin of resection. Specimen radiography is also useful in directing the pathologist to the site within the biopsy specimen that contains the suspicious lesion.

Specimen radiography can be performed using a mammography unit or an x-ray unit specifically designed for specimen radiography. Various specially designed containers are available to hold and compress the specimen and allow localization of the site of the tumor within the specimen. Comparison of the specimen radiograph with the preoperative mammogram is necessary to determine whether the lesion has been excised. This assessment must be made while the patient is still on the operating table.

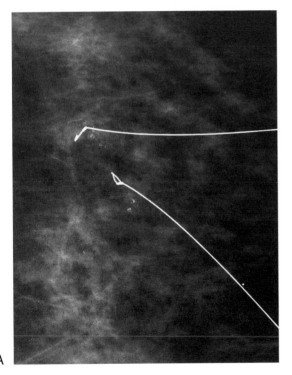

A

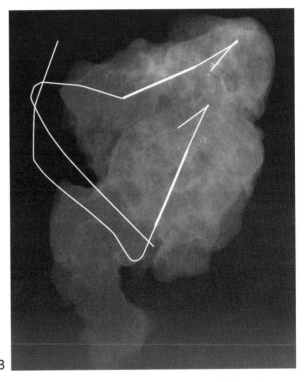

B

Fig. 3-6. More than one wire can be used to localize large lesions or multiple areas in the breast. **(A)** In this patient, two clusters of microcalcifications are present; therefore, two wires were introduced to localize both clusters. **(B)** The specimen radiograph shows that both clusters are included in the excised breast tissue and directs the pathologist to the area of tissue, which should be carefully examined histologically.

These specimens are often not analyzed by frozen section because of their small volume and the need to assess multiple sections to obtain an accurate diagnosis. Because needle localization is rarely performed as part of the definitive therapeutic procedure, histologic assessment with frozen section is rarely required at the time of biopsy.

FAILURE RATE AND COMPLICATIONS OF NEEDLE LOCALIZATION

Failure to remove a lesion at needle localization ranges from 1 to 8 percent.[7] Removal of more than one specimen may be necessary in about 20 percent of procedures. Interestingly, poor positioning of the localization wire is rarely the cause of a failed procedure. Poor communication between the surgeon and radiologist, transection of the wire intraoperatively, and migration of the wire in a fatty breast are the usual causes. If the lesion cannot be excised successfully, the surgery should be terminated. Repeat mammography after the breast has healed is indicated. If the lesion persists, a repeat needle localized biopsy should be performed.

Complications of needle localization are very rare; however, patient fainting, not a true complication, is not unusual. It has been reported in 1 percent of cases.[8] Vasovagal reactions, however, ranging from light-headedness to fainting, may occur in 7 percent of needle localizations. Because of the high level of patient anxiety during localization and the possibility of a syncopal event, either a technologist or physician should be in the room at all times during the localization procedure. Calm and confident personnel help reassure the patient. Distracting conversation with her during the procedure is often helpful. Because fainting is not rare, the room in which localizations are performed should be able to hold a stretcher on which the patient can lie down. Ampuls of ammonia also should be kept in the room, and personnel performing these procedures should be competent in treating vasovagal reactions.

Extreme pain is an unusual event during needle localization and has been reported in less than 1 percent of cases. Local anesthetic may be useful in these women. Prolonged bleeding is also rare.

SPECIAL SITUATIONS

Lesions seen only on one view can be localized with methods that use slight angulation of the x-ray tube and triangulation to determine the appropriate depth of the lesion.[9] This is most easily performed using stereotaxic biopsy equipment.[10] If these lesions can be identified sonographically, ultrasound-guided localization can be used. Lesions that can be identified on computed tomography (CT) also can be localized with CT. This option may be particularly helpful for lesions close to the chest wall or deep within the axilla.

Subtle lesions that are well visualized only with magnification can be localized with magnification technique. It must be remembered, however, that measurements are inaccurate with magnification, and appropriate adjustments must be made.

Needle localizations performed using digital spot imaging also produce magnified images because of the geometry of the systems. This type of imaging allows for faster localization because of the rapid availability of images after x-ray exposure is made. The time to complete these needle localizations is half that needed for procedures performed with traditional imaging. Additionally, radiation exposure is reduced by 30 to 45 percent.[11]

Women with breast augmentation prostheses who require needle localization should be warned that the localization procedure can result in rupture of the prosthesis. This possibility also should be noted on the informed consent form. In some instances, accurate localization can be accomplished by placing a mark on the skin overlying the lesion. The needle should be positioned within the breast so that it is parallel to the prosthesis, not directed toward it. Imaging is performed with the prosthesis displaced by the compression paddle, as it is during displaced routine views used during screening in these women. (Fig. 3-7).

OTHER LOCALIZATION TECHNIQUES

Sonography is a rapid and accurate needle localization method for lesions that are sonographically visible. However, a significant proportion of solid masses and almost all calcifications will not be evident with sonography. During this procedure, a hand-which approximates the position she is in during the biopsy procedure. The skin-to-lesion distance may be very short during the localization, and sufficient wire must be left outside the breast to allow for the increased skin-to-lesion distance when the patient is upright. After the localization has been performed, a mammogram should be obtained with the wire or dye in place. These films are labeled and sent to the operating room with the patient, as is the practice for procedures performed under mammographic control.

Devices for performing localization of biopsy with patients under magnetic resonance imaging (MRI) have been described. The device is necessary for lesions that are identifiable only with MRI; its applicability for other lesions has not been tested.

REFERENCES

1. Meyer JE, Sonnenfeld MR, Greenes RA, et al. Cancellation of preoperative breast localization procedures: analysis of 53 cases. Radiology 1988; 169:629–630.
2. Davis PS, Wechsler RJ, Feig SA, March DE. Migration of breast biopsy localization wire. Am J Roentgenol 1988; 150:787–788.
3. Tykka H, Castren-Persons M, Sjoblom SM, Roiha M. Pneumothorax caused by hooked wire localisation of an impalpable breast lesion detected by mammography. Breast 1993; 2:52–53.
4. Homer MJ. Transection of the localization hooked wire during breast biopsy. Am J Roentgenol 1983; 929–930.
5. Hirsch JI, Banks WL, Sullivan JS, Horsley JS. Effect of methylene blue on estrogen-receptor activity. Radiology 1989; 171:105–107.
6. Reynolds HE, Jackson VP, Musick BS. Preoperative needle localization in the breast: utility of local anesthesia. Radiology 1993; 187:503–505.
7. Alexander HR, Candela FC, Dershaw DD, Kinne DW. Needle-localized mammographic lesions: results and evolving treatment strategy. Arch Surg 1990; 125: 1441–1444.
8. Helvie MA, Ikeda DM, Adler DD. Localization and needle aspiration of breast lesions: complications in 370 cases. Am J Roentgenol 1991; 157:711–714.
9. Yagan R, Wiesen E, Bellon EM. Mammographic needle localization of lesions seen in only one view. Am J Roentgenol 1985; 144:911–916.
10. Chen HH, Bernstein JR, Paige ML, Crampton AR. Needle localization of nonpalpable breast lesions with a portable dual-grid compression system. Radiology 1989; 170:687—690.
11. Dershaw DD, Fleischman RC, Liberman L, et al. Use of digital mammography in needle localization proce-

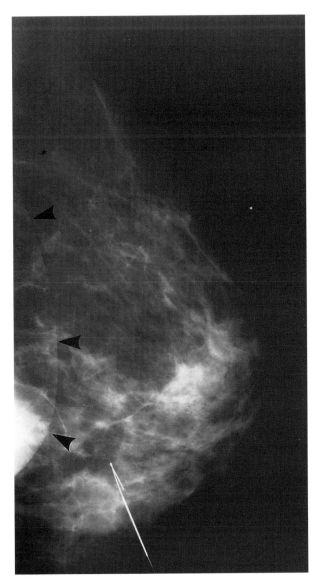

Fig. 3-7. Needle localization can be performed successfully in women with augmentation prostheses. This postlocalization image, obtained with the implant displacement technique, shows that a wire has been positioned in an area of suspicious calcifications, and the implant (*arrowheads*) is well removed from the wire. When these patients undergo localization, however, they should be informed of the possibility of implant rupture.

held, high-resolution, linear array transducer is required to perform the localization, which is performed identically to ultrasound-guided breast biopsy. The patient is localized while in the supine position,

4 PATIENT SELECTION AND CARE FOR PERCUTANEOUS BREAST BIOPSY

Ellen Shaw de Paredes

As the radiologist's role in breast imaging has expanded to include the performance of various interventional procedures, the clinical responsibility also has increased. More patients are accessing mammography services by referring themselves or requesting their own studies, and the radiologist has become responsible for managing the patient, communicating the results, and tracking the outcome.

The interventional breast imager must have knowledge about the indications and techniques for performing procedures; the selection of the best procedure to manage the patient; and the risks, limitations, and contraindications of each procedure. A preprocedural clinical assessment of the patient includes an imaging assessment, a breast-related medical history, and a limited clinical history. Discussion with the referring physician and patient is an important part of preparation for the outcome of the biopsy. Postprocedural assessment may involve a clinical visit with the patient and requires a review of her biopsy results and a determination of recommendations for further management. The time spent before and after the procedure by the radiologist is often more lengthy than the time spent in performing the technical aspects of the biopsy.

This chapter reviews the considerations for selecting patients for various types of percutaneous breast biopsy and the preprocedural and postprocedural aspects of care.

FORMS OF BIOPSY

Currently, percutaneous breast biopsies are performed for palpable and nonpalpable breast lesions that require further intervention for diagnosis. Historically, the approach to palpable breast masses began with excisional biopsy; this approach is still the standard approach used by many surgeons. Later, the use of 14-gauge Tru-cut-type core needles afforded a percutaneous approach to diagnose a palpable breast lesion. This technique was replaced in the 1980s by fine needle aspiration biopsy (FNAB), the percutaneous technique of placing a "thin" needle for retrieving samples of cells from a lesion for cytologic analysis.[1] FNAB was preferable to core needle sampling because it is easier to perform, is less traumatic, and allows for multiple passes in a fanning motion within a lesion.[1]

For nonpalpable, suspicious lesions identified on mammography, excisional biopsy after a needle localization procedure has been a standard approach until recently. With the development of improved imaging techniques, including new transducers for breast ultrasound and stereotaxis for mammographic imaging, the radiologist has gained greater accuracy in targeting a nonpalpable breast lesion. FNAB was used initially[2] with stereotaxis, but has been replaced in many facilities by larger-gauge core biopsy. FNAB requires accurate targeting of the lesion, skill in sam-

37

pling and aspiration techniques, and expert cytopathology. FNAB allows for the diagnosis of cysts, fibroadenomas, lymph nodes, and carcinoma[3]; but many benign lesions do not yield specific cytologic diagnoses. With core biopsy, specific benign and malignant histologic diagnoses are made, even for lesions that are problematic with FNAB, such as various forms of fibrocystic changes.

PATIENT SELECTION

The purpose of performing a percutaneous rather than an open or excisional biopsy is to provide a diagnosis with a less invasive and less costly procedure. Selection of patients for percutaneous biopsy must consider potential management decisions for various histologic diagnoses. Percutaneous biopsy should not be used if it will merely add another step in the work-up of the patient with a breast abnormality.

With greater utilization of screening mammography, increasing numbers of biopsies are performed for nonspecific, suspicious mammographic abnormalities that are benign lesions. The positive predictive value for nonpalpable, suspicious lesions that are biopsied is in the range of 10 to 35 percent.[4] An important role of percutaneous biopsy is to confirm a benign diagnosis for lesions that are indeterminate by mammography and to avoid surgical biopsy of these lesions.

Percutaneous biopsy also is used to diagnose a highly suspicious lesion as malignant, thus avoiding a two-step surgical procedure for diagnosis and treatment. Lesions that are considered probably benign (i.e., likelihood of malignancy less than 2 percent[5]) and for which an early mammographic follow-up would be recommended should be handled as such. In general, percutaneous biopsy should not be substituted for early mammographic follow-up, but should be recommended for the evaluation of lesions amenable to excisional biopsy.[6] For patients who are extremely anxious about early follow-up or who may not be able to obtain a follow-up mammogram, percutaneous biopsy may be substituted for early mammographic follow-up.[7]

A prebiopsy review of the patient's imaging studies must be performed to determine the best type of biopsy for the patient and the type of lesion, the form of guidance (stereotaxic, mammographic, sonograph-

ic) and the plan for approaching the lesion. Ideally, this imaging assessment should be conducted before the patient's arrival in the department so that procedure rooms can be used most effectively and needed equipment is available.

In conjunction with the actual review of mammography and other imaging studies, the radiologist also should review the patient's breast-related history that might affect the ultimate management decisions. Patients with known high risk factors, prior breast cancer, or premalignant conditions in either breast may have a higher level of suspicion attributed to an indeterminate lesion. All imaging must be completed before performing an interventional procedure. A complete diagnostic work-up, including spot compression or magnification views or ultrasound if necessary, must be performed before recommending any type of biopsy.

Lesions most amenable to diagnosis by FNAB are (1) probable cysts that are equivocal or complex on ultrasound, (2) probable fibroadenomas (well-circumscribed, solid masses), (3) probable enlarged or abnormal intramammary lymph nodes, and (4) probable carcinomas (spiculated masses or malignant microcalcifications).[3,8,9] Problematic lesions on FNAB are (1) lesions that are relatively acellular (fibrosis, sclerotic fibroadenomas), (2) radial scars because of the atypical appearance of the cells on cytology, and (3) fibrocystic lesions that present as indistinct masses or microcalcifications. Indeterminate mammographic lesions may need to be excised when a nonspecific cytologic result is rendered. Therefore, FNAB may not benefit patients with noncystic fibrocystic conditions and may just add another step in the patient's work-up and management. As with core biopsy, a highly suspicious mammographic finding with a benign FNAB result warrants excisional biopsy.[3,10]

The majority of nonpalpable mammographic lesions are amenable to core biopsy. These lesions include (1) well-defined solid masses, (2) indistinct or spiculated masses, and (3) clustered microcalcifications.[11-13] Lesions that are of relatively low suspicion in the indeterminate group of nonpalpable abnormalities and those that are of high suspicion are well suited for evaluation by percutaneous core biopsy.[11-13] For a relatively low-suspicion lesion, if the diagnosis on core biopsy is benign, excisional biopsy can be avoided, and mammographic follow-up can be obtained.[14] For a high-suspicion mammographic lesion with a positive biopsy result, definitive treatment can be planned.

Percutaneous biopsy is particularly advantageous in the evaluation of multiple clusters of suspicious microcalcifications or of multiple malignant-appearing masses in the same breast. If two or more lesions are malignant, the patient is not a candidate for breast conservation and mastectomy should be performed without the need for further biopsy or excision of the lesion. For a single lesion in which breast conservation rather than mastectomy would be performed, a presurgical diagnosis of carcinoma can allow for a segmental resection and axillary node dissection as a single procedure rather than as two separate surgical interventions. Some surgeons, however, may argue that a percutaneous biopsy is superfluous because an excisional biopsy is necessary to evaluate tumor margins before the node dissection and re-excision are performed.[11]

Problematic lesions for stereotaxic core biopsy include those that are difficult to target or those that may be problematic for diagnosis (Table 4-1). Targeting problems can be related to the position of the lesion in the breast or to the indistinctness of the lesion. Lesions located far posteriorly near the chest wall are difficult to pull forward enough to keep the area in position for accurate targeting and biopsy. The upright stereotaxic attachments are somewhat more flexible than the prone table units in terms of positioning the patient with a very posterior lesion. On the prone units, the thickness of the edge of the table adds to the inability to visualize a very posterior lesion, whereas the edge of the compression plate on the upright unit is the limiting factor for positioning. In either case, on most types of units a lesion near the chest wall is difficult to position and to maintain in position for adequate biopsy.[12,13] If visible under ultrasound, these lesions may be more amenable to sonographically guided biopsy.

Table 4-1. Problematic Lesions
for Percutaneous Biopsy

Lesions less than 5 mm
Fine, scattered microcalcifications
Indistinct densities
Architectural distortion/possible radial scar
Posterior lesions near the chest wall
Lesions in the axillary tail
Very superficial lesions

Other problems related to lesion position include a very superficial[13] lesion in which one may not be able to insert the needle proximal to the lesion and to allow for the needle excursion without bypassing the mass. Lesions located high in the axillary tail are also difficult to maintain in position for adequate targeting and biopsy.

A very small lesion (< 5 mm) might not be considered appropriate for excisional biopsy for two reasons. First, targeting must be extremely accurate to biopsy the lesion. More important, with successful targeting and biopsy, the entire lesion may be removed; if biopsy shows malignancy, the actual site of the lesion may not be visible for excision.[15,16]

Indistinct masses or areas of asymmetry or very fine microcalcifications may be difficult to image stereotaxically,[13,17] even with digital imaging, and may not be targeted adequately. Because a grid is not used for stereotaxic imaging, the contrast is decreased compared with routine mammography. Additionally, compression of the area of interest is less than that with mammography, so that imaging of soft tissue densities within parenchyma can be hampered significantly. These factors affect the stereotaxic imaging and accurate targeting of mammographic abnormalities, particularly of indistinct densities and fine microcalcifications.

Lesions that can be identified on ultrasound and that are suspicious enough to warrant an intervention are amenable to percutaneous biopsy with ultrasound guidance. Ultrasound can provide fast and easy access for visualization and biopsy of non-palpable lesions without the need for ionizing radiation. The choice of whether to use ultrasound or stereotaxis for a mass seen in both modalities is often related to the preference and skill of the radiologist. With ultrasound, the biopsy can be observed and documented in real time.[18] Great care must be used when directing the needle, however, to avoid placing the needle tip into the chest wall. This factor is particularly critical with core biopsy, where the distance of the throw of the needle and the relationship of the position of the prefire needle tip to the lesion and the chest wall must be considered carefully. Especially with very posterior lesions ultrasound guidance may be difficult, and an approach parallel to the chest wall is maintained[19] to avoid complications.

Indeterminate lesions that are highly suspicious so that one may not be satisfied with relying on a benign biopsy result are problematic because of histologic/mammographic correlation.[11] These lesions may be evaluated better with needle localization and excisional biopsy.

A particularly difficult lesion to diagnose by core biopsy is radial scar.[11–13] The pathologist relies on the distinctive architecture and the cellular features to make the diagnosis of radial scar. Because core biopsy is a sampling type of biopsy, the spokewheel architecture of the radial scar is not usually perceived.[11] Radial scar can potentially cause a false-positive or suspicious reading on the pathologic analysis. For these reasons, areas of architectural distortion that have a radial scar appearance should be excised, not biopsied percutaneously.[3,11,17]

Another problematic lesion for core biopsy is a loose group of microcalcifications.[6,11,12] To biopsy an area of microcalcifications, one targets specific calcifications in the area. With a loosely arranged group of calcifications covering a large area, targeting and adequate sampling may be compromised unless one makes multiple skin incisions and biopsies throughout the entire region.

Clinical considerations for selecting patients for percutaneous biopsy include an assessment of factors that might increase the risk of the infrequent but potential complications of bleeding or infection. Small, superficial hematomas may be identified in as many as 40 percent of cases,[13] but larger significant hematomas are uncommon with FNAB or core biopsy.[20–22] A prebiopsy clinical assessment of the patient should be conducted, either at the time of scheduling or before the procedure (Fig. 4-1). A technologist or nurse may conduct the interview and document the history on a questionnaire that becomes part of the patient's record. Routine preoperative blood work-up is not usually performed unless there is a clinical indication of potential prolonged bleeding.[6]

Possible causes for prolonged bleeding must be identified and either corrected or considered as a potential contraindication to percutaneous biopsy, particularly large-gauge core biopsy. Anticoagulant therapy is a contraindication to percutaneous biopsy.[17] Patients on warfarin sodium (Coumadin) therapy should discontinue use of the anticoagulant with advice from their physician, and clotting studies should be performed before a percutaneous biopsy is performed. Patients who take aspirin or nonsteroidal anti-inflammatory drugs routinely also should ideally discontinue use of these medications for at least 48 hours before the procedure.

Medical causes of prolonged bleeding include clotting disorders and liver disease. If the patient is known to have either of these conditions, preoperative clotting times should be obtained; if clotting times are elevated, the risk of bleeding or significant hematoma increases.

Infections after FNAB are relatively rare.[23] Various reports of core biopsy series also have found a low risk of postbiopsy infection.[13,24] From needle localization and excisional biopsy series, Rappaport et al.[25] found postoperative infections in 11 of 144 patients. These infections were thought to be related most often to the presence of surgical drains.

Breast surgery is considered a clean procedure in general and does not require prophylactic antibiotics. The role of prophylactic antibiotics for breast procedures is unclear, and studies on the role of prophylaxis for percutaneous biopsy have not been reported. The same principles for antibiotic use should apply to percutaneous breast biopsy as for breast surgical procedures, but one must emphasize the need to maintain sterile techniques. For core biopsy, the skin under the aperture, the needle, and the needle guide are sterile; and the remainder of the field is nonsterile. While performing the procedure, one must be diligent in handling the needle and the skin surface to avoid contamination.

Some authors[26,27] have suggested the use of prophylactic antibiotics for breast surgeries and have reported a decrease in postoperative infections. Platt et al.[26] reported 48 percent fewer postoperative infections in patients who had herniorrhaphy or breast surgery and who received perioperative antibiotic prophylaxis. In patients who are immunocompromised or who have a history of insulin-dependent diabetes mellitus, prophylaxis before percutaneous biopsy should be considered.

Postoperative infections are often caused by *Staphylococcus aureus.*[28] Antibiotic prophylaxis can include cephalosporins[27] (cefonicid, 1 g IV 30 minutes before the procedure) or penicillins with coverage for *Staphylococcus.*

Prophylactic antibiotics are administered to prevent bacterial endocarditis in patients with a history of rheumatic fever or prosthetic heart valves. These

1)   Do you have a history of the following:

-    Diabetes mellitus?   YES____   NO____

-    Liver disease?   YES____   NO____

-    Bleeding problems?   YES____   NO____

-    Rheumatic fever?   YES____   NO____

-    Artificial heart valve?   YES____   NO____

2)   Do you take anticoagulants (blood thinners)?   YES____   NO____

3)   Do you take aspirin daily?   YES____   NO____

When was your last dose of aspirin?_____

4)   Do you take prophylactic antibiotics before surgical or dental procedures?

YES____   NO____

5)   Do you have any allergies?   YES____   NO____

If yes, please describe:_____

_____

Fig. 4-1. Preoperative patient assessment for percutaneous breast biopsy.

antibiotics are recommended when these patients undergo dental or surgical procedures in the upper respiratory tract[29] or certain procedures in the genitourinary and gastrointestinal tracts. Although some procedures, including percutaneous liver biopsy, rarely have been subsequently associated with infective endocarditis, prophylaxis may be administered for patients who are at particularly high risk (e.g., with prosthetic heart valves).[29]

The Committee on Rheumatic Fever and Infective Endocarditis[29] has recognized that "practitioners must exercise their clinical judgment in determining the duration and choice of antibiotics when special circumstances apply." Because the actual sterile field during stereotactic biopsy is quite small and because of the nonsterile components of the equipment near the field, one might consider the use of prophylaxis in patients with a history of rheumatic heart or valvular prosthesis.

The need for and type of antibiotic for prophylaxis in these patients, however, has not been defined.

Before the percutaneous biopsy is performed, informed consent should be obtained. The patient should be informed of the reason for performing the biopsy, the expected procedure, the risk of bleeding or infection, and potential outcomes. The patient should understand that she may need a repeat biopsy if the specimen is unsatisfactory and may need an excision of the lesion if the pathologic findings are suspicious. The preoperative clinical assessment should be reviewed before performing the procedure.

POSTPROCEDURE ASSESSMENT

After an FNAB, the skin should be cleaned with alcohol and a Band-Aid applied to the puncture site. Ice may be applied to the breast if bleeding occurred during the biopsy. In most cases, however, no ice pack is necessary, although some have recommended its routine application.

After core biopsy, manual compression is applied for 5 to 10 minutes to avoid a hematoma. The skin should be cleaned with sterile water or alcohol. The skin incision is apposed with a Steri-strip, and antibiotic ointment may be applied at the incision site. A Band-Aid or a 4 × 4 gauze is placed over the steristrip, and the patient is advised to keep the steristrip in place for 48 hours. An ice pack is applied to the site for 30 minutes, and the patient is advised to re-apply the ice pack after 1 hour, and again later if necessary. Nonaspirin-containing analgesics may be used for pain.

The patient is instructed to observe the breast for any sign of bleeding or infection, and she is given information on whom to contact if this should occur. A small or moderate-sized hematoma is indicated by fullness at the puncture site with bruising. Small hematomas gradually resolve without intervention. A large hematoma may be a tender mass and require surgical evacuation.

Signs of mastitis include pain, erythema, purulent drainage from the biopsy site or nipple, skin thickening or swelling, increased skin temperature over the breast, and fever.[30] If postbiopsy mastitis or abscess is suspected, culture and sensitivity testing of an aspirate can be performed. Most infections are produced by *S. aureus* or anaerobes; a cephalosporin or a drug such as amoxicillin/clavulanate potassium (Augmentin)[30] can be used to treat mastitis.

The patient also is told how she will receive the biopsy results. The referring physician or radiologist may provide the results of the biopsy to the patient; if the radiologist does not provide the results directly to the patient, it is critical that she communicate to the referring physician the biopsy result and the overall recommendation based on the mammographic and cytologic or histologic findings. The radiologist also must assure the patient that the referring physician will provide the results.

If the radiologist provides the results to the patient, the patient may be asked to return for a wound check[6] and to be given the results in person. This approach is especially important when the biopsy demonstrates a malignancy. In consideration of the patient, some do not give results over the phone to the patient if cancer is found.

Regardless of who will provide the biopsy results to the patient, postprocedural instructions should include the phone number of the breast imaging facility to call if she has any clinical problems, questions, or has not received her biopsy results by an indicated period of time. If the results are benign and the radiologist recommends an early follow-up mammogram in 6 months, the patient may be scheduled for her follow-up appointment. Both written and verbal postprocedural instructions are helpful in clarifying the preceding points to the patient (Fig. 4-2).

SUMMARY

One of the most important components of a percutaneous biopsy is the mammographic and pathologic correlation of findings and planning the management of the patient. The level of suspicion of the mammographic lesion, the accuracy of the targeting of the lesions, and the confirmation of microcalcifications in the specimen for calcified lesions must be considered carefully and correlated with the cytologic or histologic findings. If the level of mammographic suspicion is high and the biopsy result is benign, excision of the lesion should be performed.

- Apply ice to the breast for 30 minutes three times on the day of your procedure to relieve swelling and bruising.

- You may use Tylenol (two tablets) every four to six hours for pain if needed.

- You may return to work after the procedure, but do not perform any strenuous activities for 24 to 48 hours.

- You may remove the bandage tomorrow morning, but keep the thin strip of tape in place for two days.

- You may notice bruising in the area of the biopsy. This will usually clear in five to seven days.

- If you notice any bleeding, drainage, excessive swelling, pain, redness, or heat around the biopsy area please call

_____.

The final results of your biopsy are usually available in two to three working days.

_____ will contact you with the results. If you have not heard your results within five working days, please call _____.

Fig. 4-2. Postbreast biopsy patient instructions.

REFERENCES

1. Donegan WL. Evaluation of a palpable breast mass. New Engl J Med 1992; 327:937–942.
2. Svane G. Stereotactic needle biopsy of nonpalpable breast lesions. Acta Radiol 1983; 24:284–288.
3. Shaw de Paredes E. Stereotactic needle biopsies: FNA. In: Syllabus 26th National Conference on Breast Cancer. American College of Radiology, Washington, DC 1994;14–15.
4. Shaw de Paredes E. Atlas of Film-Screen Mammography. 2nd Ed. Williams & Wilkins, Philadelphia, 1992.
5. Sickles EA. Periodic mammographic follow-up of probably benign lesions: results in 3,184 consecutive cases. Radiology 1991; 179:463–468.
6. Meyer JE. Value of large core biopsy of occult breast lesions. Am J Roentgenol 1992; 158:991–992.
7. Sickles EA, Parker SH. Appropriate role of core biopsy in the management of probably benign lesions. Radiology 1993; 188:315.
8. Hirschowitz SL. Stereotactic needle biopsies: FNA. In: Syllabus 26th National Conference on Breast Cancer. American College of Radiology, Washington, DC 1994;11–13.
9. Dowlatshahi K, Yaremko ML, Kluskins LF, Jokich PM. Nonpalpable breast lesions: findings of stereotactic needle-core biopsy and fine needle aspiration cytology. Radiology 1991; 181:745–750.
10. Lofgren M, Andersson I, Lindholm K. Stereotactic fine-needle aspiration for cytologic diagnosis of nonpalpa-

ble breast lesions. Am J Roentgenol 1990; 154: 1191–1195.

11. Evans P, Oberman H. Stereotactic needle biopsies: core and FNA. In: Syllabus 26th National Conference on Breast Cancer. American College of Radiology 1994;9–10.

12. Parker SH, Lovin JD, Jobe WE, et al. Nonpalpable breast lesions: stereotactic automated large-core biopsies. Radiology 1991; 180:403–407.

13. Sullivan DC. Needle core biopsy of mammographic lesions. Am J Roentgenol 1994; 162:601–608.

14. Gisvold JJ, Goellner JR, Grant CS, et al: Breast biopsy: a comparative study of stereotaxically guided core and excisional techniques. Am J Roentgenol 1994; 162: 815–820.

15. Dronkers DJ. Stereotaxic core biopsy of breast lesions. Radiology 1992; 183:631–634.

16. Jackson VP, Reynolds HE. Stereotaxic needle-core biopsy and fine-needle aspiration cytologic evaluation of nonpalpable breast lesions. Radiology 1991; 181:633–634.

17. Bird RE. Image guided needle biopsy of the breast. In: Syllabus 26th National Conference on Breast Cancer. American College of Radiology, 1994;25–27.

18. Fornage BD, Coan JD, David CL. Ultrasound-guided needle biopsy of the breast and other interventional procedures. Radiol Clin North Am 1992; 30:167–185.

19. Parker SH, Jobe WE, Dennis MA, et al. US-guided automated large-core breast biopsy. Radiology 1993; 187:507–511.

20. Caines JS, McPhee MD, Konok GP, Wright BA. Stereotaxic needle core biopsy of breast lesions using a regular mammographic table with an adaptable stereotaxic device. Am J Roentgenol 1994; 163:317–321.

21. Parker SH. When is core biopsy really core? Radiology 1992; 185:641–642.

22. Hann L, Ducatman BS, Wang HH, et al. Nonpalpable breast lesions: evaluation by means of fine-needle aspiration cytology. Radiology 1989; 171:373–376.

23. Shabot MM, Goldberg IM, Schick P, et al. Aspiration cytology is superior to tru-cut needle biopsy in establishing the diagnosis of clinically suspicious breast masses. Ann Surg 1982; 196:122–126.

24. Pezner RD, Lorant JA, Terz J, et al. Wound-healing complications following biopsy of the irradiated breast. Arch Surg 1992; 127:321–324.

25. Rappaport W, Thompson S, Wong R, et al. Complications associated with needle localization biopsy of the breast. Surg Gynecol Obstet 1991; 172:303–306.

26. Platt R, Zaleznik DF, Hopkins CC, et al. Perioperative antibiotic prophylaxis for herniorrhaphy and breast surgery. N Engl J Med 1990; 322:153–160.

27. Platt R, Zucker JR, Zaleznik DF, et al: Prophylaxis against wound infection following herniorrhaphy or breast surgery. J Infect Dis 1992; 166:556–560.

28. Nichols RL. Surgical wound infection. Am J Med 1991; 91(suppl 3B):3B54S–3B64S.

29. Shulman ST, Amren DP, Bisno AL, et al. Prevention of bacterial endocarditis. Circulation 1984; 70:1123A–1127A.

30. Giamarellou H, Soulis M, Antoniadou A, Gogas J. Periareolar nonpuerperal breast infection: treatment of 38 cases. Clin Infect Dis 1994; 18:73–76.

5 EQUIPMENT CONSIDERATIONS: STEREOTAXIC AND DIGITAL SYSTEMS

Laurie Fajardo

Distinguishing between malignant and benign breast lesions may be difficult based on mammography alone. Histologic evaluation is often necessary. Dedicated prone stereotaxic mammography equipment was first described in 1977.[1] Recently, percutaneous stereotaxic breast needle biopsy has been introduced clinically in the United States as a viable alternative to surgical excisional breast biopsy. This radiologic interventional procedure can be performed with diagnostic accuracy equal to surgical excisional breast biopsy, is associated with less patient morbidity, and significantly reduces health care costs related to diagnosing nonpalpable breast lesions. Additionally, common postsurgical mammographic findings, such as architectural distortion due to scarring or postoperative seroma, are not encountered after stereotaxic needle biopsy.[2] As an efficacious alternative to surgical biopsy, we and others advocate using mammography-guided needle biopsy to diagnose nonpalpable breast lesions.[2–6]

Radiologists planning to begin a percutaneous breast biopsy program must make several decisions regarding the way in which biopsies will be performed. The utility of core biopsy and fine needle aspiration cytology is discussed in the next three chapters. The efficacy of sonographically guided biopsy is reviewed in Chapter 10. Details of stereotaxic biopsy are covered in Chapter 9. This chapter is designed to assist the radiologist in choosing among various types of stereotaxic equipment that are cur-

rently commercially available. Additionally, digital imaging, which can be purchased as part of some stereotaxic equipment, is discussed.

STEREOTAXIC BREAST BIOPSY SYSTEMS

Several manufacturers market stereotaxic devices, which in general are of two basic types: the so-called "add-on" or upright units and the prone, dedicated stereotaxic biopsy systems. Both types of units provide accurate needle placement for fine needle aspiration biopsy (FNAB) and large-gauge core needle biopsy.

The "add-on" or upright devices are designed to attach to existing mammography units (Fig. 5-1). These units offer the advantages of low cost ($35,000 to $40,000), the ability to use the system in a smaller sized interventional mammography suite, the ability to use the mammography unit for standard breast imaging when the stereotaxic device is not attached, and the ability to biopsy deep breast lesions and axillary lymph nodes. Deep lesions and axillary masses are sometimes not amenable to evaluation by the prone stereotaxic systems because of the unavoidable distance between the lesion and the biopsy device created by the intervening table. Disadvantages of "add-on" stereotaxic breast biopsy devices include the ability of the patient to view the biopsy procedure as it is being performed, which sometimes

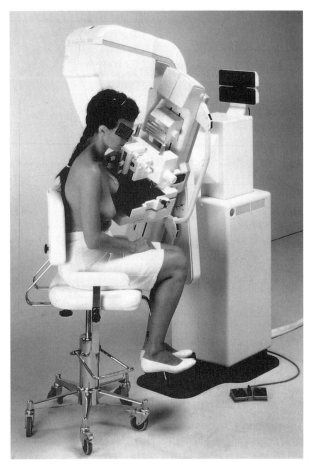

Fig. 5-1. An upright, add-on stereotaxic biopsy unit. The patient must maintain the sitting position during the biopsy, and she can watch the radiologist during the procedure. (Courtesy of General Electric, Milwaukee, Wisconsin.)

results in vasovagal reactions (1 to 5 percent) and the relatively small working space for the interventional mammographer performing biopsy procedures. This disadvantage may be particularly limiting during core biopsy procedures, which use bulkier equipment than FNABs.

Dedicated, prone stereotaxic devices offer the conveniences of greater working space for the interventionalist and a reduced incidence of vasovagal reactions due to prone, rather than upright, positioning for procedures. In addition, the biopsy equipment and needles are beneath the system table and are not visualized by the patient during the procedure. While dedicated, prone stereotaxic systems are consider-

ably more expensive ($140,000 to over $200,000 for those with digital imaging capability), they have become extremely popular in clinical, radiologic, and surgical practices during the last 5 years. Because such systems cannot be used for routine breast imaging, they require the performance of a minimum number of interventional procedures to justify the purchase cost.

The two major manufacturers of dedicated, prone stereotaxic breast biopsy systems are Fischer Imaging Corporation (Fischer Mammotest; Thornton, CO) and LORAD (LORAD Medical Systems; Danbury, CT) (Fig. 5-2). Both systems allow an unrestricted working area, out of the patient's view, for performing stereotaxic breast needle biopsy. Each of these two systems, however, has different design features. To adequately use a Fischer unit, the room must be large enough to position the unit outward from the corner of the room or within the center of a room. That is, the radiologist must be able to access both sides of the table to perform biopsies on the right or left breast from a variety of approaches. Further, access to the breast for needle biopsy using the Fischer system is limited to less than 360 degrees. The LORAD unit can be positioned lengthwise against a wall in an interventional suite, which requires considerably less room for its housing. Further, 360-degree access is afforded by this machine because patients can be positioned from either end of the table.

There are also differences with respect to the approaches used for by the manufacturers for calculating the x, y, and z, coordinates for the location of the lesion within the breast. The Fischer Imaging System uses polar coordinates for targeting, whereas the LORAD systems uses rectangular or Cartesian coordinates. Polar coordinates are based on measurements of degrees or radian, whereas polar coordinates use standard horizontal (x), vertical (y), and depth (z) measurements. Although Cartesian coordinate systems are intuitively easier to understand and master, both manufacturers have developed computerized, automated mechanisms for computing calculations and accurately positioning biopsy needle tips at the breast skin surface. The polar coordinate system is equivalent to the Cartesian system so long as no error in localizing a breast lesion occurs. However, if the interventional mammographer introduces error (i.e., inability to definitively target a

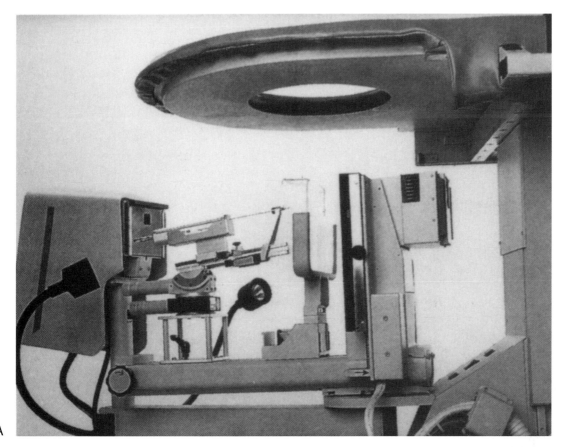

A

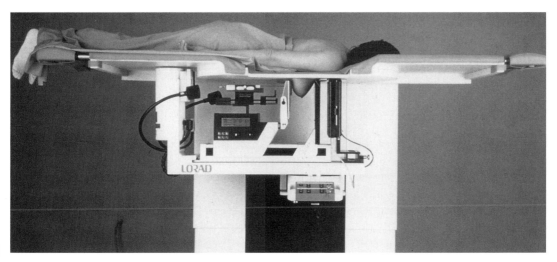

B

Fig. 5-2. (A) Fischer dedicated prone stereotaxic unit. The hole for breast placement is at the end of the table, so that the patient's head must always be directed toward that end. (Courtesy of Fischer Corporation, Thornton, CO.) **(B)** LORAD dedicated prone stereotaxic unit. The hole for breast placement is in the center of the table, which allows the patient's feet to be placed at either end. This make a caudal-cranial approach possible. (Courtesy of LORAD Corporation, Danbury, CT.) *(Figure continues.)*

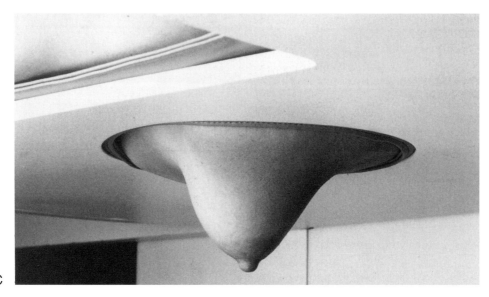

C

Fig. 5-2. *(Continued)*. **(C)** The breast is dependent during the biopsy procedure, and the table separates the patient from the radiologist. (Courtesy of LORAD Corporation, Danbury, CT.)

lesion in the same spot on both the +15- and −15-degree images), and if the abnormality is located near the edge of the 5 × 5 cm biopsy window, error will be greater for the polar coordinate system than for the Cartesian system.

STEREOTAXIC BIOPSY SYSTEM IMAGING RECEPTORS

For stereotaxic breast imaging, two systems are currently used: screen-film imaging systems and digital, charge-coupled device (CCD) imaging systems. Both systems are available on the currently marketed prone, dedicated stereotaxic breast biopsy systems. Most "add-on," upright stereotaxic devices, however, utilize screen-film receptors. With digital imaging systems, stereotaxic images are available within 3 to 5 seconds after an exposure. Having images in digital format also facilitates fast and accurate lesion targeting, with the use of image display computer software.

The two dedicated, prone biopsy systems differ in the type of screen-film system offered for stereotaxic imaging. LORAD uses a reciprocating ("Bucky") grid with a 5:1 grid ratio and a grid density of 33 lines/cm. Fischer uses a stationary grid with a grid ratio of 3.5:1 and a grid density of 80 lines/cm. The latter system is limited to using a stationary grid because the x-ray tube and image receptor do not rotate together when performing stereotaxic imaging. Rather, the x-ray tube rotates 15 degrees to the right or left, whereas the image receptor is oriented at a 75-degree angle to the x-ray tube.

The CCD cameras currently used for digital stereotaxic imaging acquisition use either lens-coupled or fiberoptic-coupled CCDs as the image receptor and offer several advantages over film-based stereotaxic imaging.[7] First, the process of image acquisition is decoupled from that of display. This means that the gray-scale of CCD-acquired images can be manipulated after acquisition to maximize the contrast and lesion conspicuity. Postacquisition manipulation of image data is not possible with film. Second, because CCD images are displayed on a CRT monitor in 3 to 5 seconds after an exposure, the placement of a biopsy needle can be quickly confirmed before sampling. Because digital stereotaxic systems allow a breast needle biopsy to be performed in "pseudoreal" time, they offer considerable efficiency related to time savings over film-based systems that use routine image processing. Other advantages include wide image latitude, increased low contrast resolution, increased signal-to-noise ratio, and the ability to directly digitize images. Digital stereotaxic breast imaging systems are inferior in spatial resolution with respect to film-based systems (5 to 9 lp/mm versus 15 lp/mm).[7] Digital systems also decrease the radiation dose per exposure by one-third to one-half that required by film-screen systems.[8]

The Fischer Imaging digital camera utilizes fiberoptic coupling to the CCD receptor (Fig. 5-3A) and has better spatial resolution (7 to 8 lp/mm) as compared to that of the lens-coupled LORAD system (5 to 6 lp/mm) (Fig. 5-3B). The design of the LORAD lens coupled CCD camera, however, enables it to gather considerably more light photons from an exposure, yielding a significantly better contrast resolution.[9] Spatial resolution is important when imaging microcalcifications, whereas contrast resolution is most important when imaging masses, low density lesions, or breast abnormalities that are obscured by overlying radiodense parenchyma.

STEREOTAXIC LOCALIZATION

Stereotaxic devices take advantage of the principle of triangulation, and calculations are based on simple trigonometric equations. Calculations of the amount of deviation of a lesion on two views, obtained 30 degrees apart, allows precise determination of a breast lesion location in three dimensions.[10] Stereotaxic views are acquired with x-ray beams directed at +15 and −15 degrees relative to a line perpendicular to the image receptor. The x horizontal location of the lesion when approached from the 0-degree or perpendicular ray (the approximate line of approach of the biopsy needle) is the average of the x locations of the lesion on the two stereotactic views. The y (vertical) location of the lesion is the same in both views. The z location (or depth) of the lesion is determined by the amount of parallax shift from one view to the other. The parallax

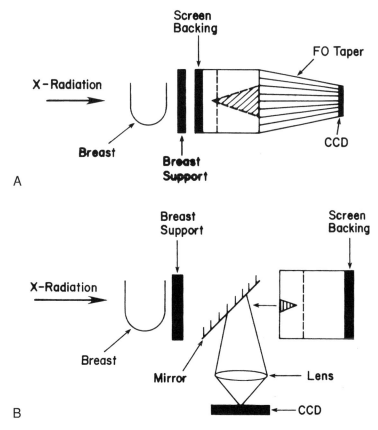

Fig. 5-3. (A) Schematic of the Fischer fiberoptic CCD digital stereotaxic breast imaging system. **(B)** Schematic of the LORAD lens coupled CCD digital stereotaxic breast imaging system.

shift is measured relative to reference markers that automatically appear on each image from small holes that are drilled into the stereotaxic breast compression device. The shift in lesion position from one stereotaxic view to the other, measured relative to the reference markers in each image, is:

$$X_s = X_{ps} - X_{rs}$$

where X_{ps} is the shift in position of the center of the lesion from one image to another and X_{rs} is the shift in the position of the reference marker from one image to another. Thus, X_s is the shift of the lesion relative to the reference markers on the +15-degree view to the −15-degree view. The distance of the lesion from the back breast support, Z_d, is given by

$$Z_d = \frac{X_s}{2\tan(15°)} = (1.866)Z_d$$

From this equation, needle insertion depth is determined. Figure 5-4 illustrates the mathematical approach to calculating the x, y, and z coordinates by either screen-film or digital imaging techniques.

ACCEPTANCE TESTING OF STEREOTAXIC BREAST BIOPSY SYSTEMS

The purchase of a stereotaxic breast biopsy unit is a three-step process: vendor identification, equipment evaluation, and acceptance testing. Identifying a vendor who will provide reliable customer support and service is an important first evaluation. The next step is to assess the imager's performance and specifications based on its medical physics data. If sufficient data are not available, a medical physicist should evaluate the components themselves, as described below. The final step is to require a vigorous acceptance test to ensure that the manufacturer's specifications have been met *before* final payment.

Upright or "add-on" stereotaxic units can be tested easily by using conventional mammography procedures and a standard stereotaxic localization phantom for assessing needle placement accuracy.[11,12] Prone units, however, are more difficult to assess because of the under-table tube configuration. Additionally, there are important design differences between conventional

mammographic units utilizing "add-on" stereotaxic equipment and the prone biopsy units. Further, the design of the two commercial dedicated prone stereotaxic mammography systems differ, such that the acceptance testing needed will vary by manufacturer.

Most quality assurance tests recommended by the American College of Radiology[12] are suitable for evaluating stereotaxic systems. Additional tests are needed, however, to ensure stereotaxic accuracy.[13] Acceptance testing of the Fischer stereotaxic biopsy system is easier than the LORAD system in some respects because the biopsy device holder can be completely removed from the system. Additionally, the Fischer system is equipped with a light that demarcates the x-ray field to allow testing equipment to be more easily positioned. However, the fixed grid and polar coordinate system used for stereotaxic calculations by the Fischer system require special testing[13] (see below). Variations from the usual quality assurance/acceptance test for conventional mammography units that are necessary for dedicated prone units are described below.

Focal Spot Testing

A 0.5-degree star pattern can be used for measuring the focal spot size of prone stereotaxic systems. The star pattern must be positioned carefully to match the magnification to the nominal focal spot size in order to capture a 0.3-mm nominal focal spot. The star pattern should be placed so that magnification is no more than × 3. Positioning of the star pattern is somewhat challenging on the LORAD system because of the lack of a light-demarcating system. Because the LORAD unit has a higher output than the Fischer unit, a 1-cm thick rectangular piece of Plexiglas may be attached to the star test pattern when measurements are made. For measuring the focal spot size of the Fischer unit, the light field can be used to guide positioning to achieve the correct magnification. The film imaging receptor should be placed in front of the Fischer system's grid rather than in the cassette tunnel because the grid will produce Moire patterns on the star image. For testing the focal spot size of either system, film should be used for imaging because the digital format on both systems is of insufficient resolution to test the effective focal spot sizes. A pinhole or slit image of the focal

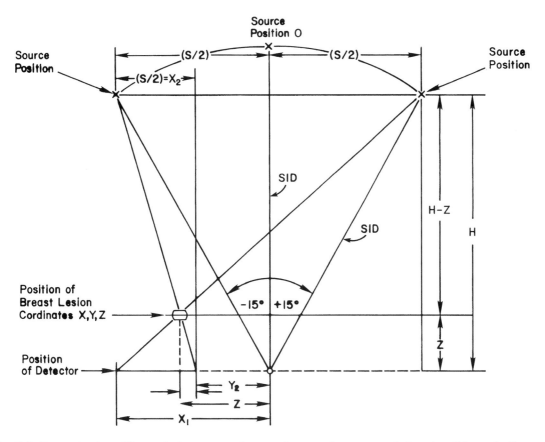

Fig. 5-4. Determination of breast lesion x, y, and z coordinates using stereotaxic imaging. Schematic diagram illustrates the geometry for calculating the x, y, and z coordinates for a lesion within the breast from the coordinates of the stereotaxic image projections x_1, y_1 and x_2, y_2. Determination of lesion coordinates by screen-film imaging technique:

$$Z = [H (X_1 - X_2)] / [S + (X_1 - X_2)]$$

$$X = X_2 + Z [S/2 - X_2] / H$$

$$Y = Y_1 (H - Z) / H = Y_2 (H - Z) / H$$

Determination of object coordinates with digital imaging methods:

$$Z = [H (n_{x,p,1} - n_{x,p,2}) \cdot d_p \cdot t_r] / [S + (n_{x,p,1} - n_{x,p,2}) \cdot d_p \cdot t_r]$$

$$X = (n_{x,p,2}) \cdot d_p \cdot t_r) + Z [(S/2) - (n_{x,p,2} \cdot d_p \cdot t_r)] / H$$

$$Y = [n_{x,p,1} \cdot d_p \cdot t_r) (H - Z)] / H = [(n_{y,p,2}) \cdot d_p \cdot t_r) (H-Z)]/H$$

H = distance between the x-ray source and detector

S = distance between source positions for +15- and −15-degree stereotaxic images.

d_p = pixel size

t_r = fiberoptic taper ratio

n = "pixel address."

spot should be attempted only if the procedure can be accomplished using a digital imaging receptor.

mR/mAs, kVp, HVL, Output Linearity

Similar to testing conventional mammography equipment, these tests require positioning an ion chamber or kVp meter in the x-ray field. It is important to note, however, that the limited field-of-view of stereotaxic units allows the manufacturers to use large anode angles on the prone systems. This increases the heel effect over that found with conventional mammography units and, as a result, inaccurate measurements can result if the ion chamber is centered more than 2 cm below the chest wall edge of the imaging device. Similarly, differences in the expected HVL may be seen because the beam in the heel of the anode is filtered by the anode material.[13]

Dose

Although stereotaxic breast biopsy procedures are considered diagnostic or therapeutic rather than screening procedures, dose measurements are useful for both acceptance testing and for monitoring the unit over time. Expert physicists feel that calculating exposure from the mAs required by the American College of Radiology (ACR) mammography phantom and the calculated mR/mAs is justified so long as the output linearity of a particular system is within 5 percent.[13] As a general rule, dose measurement on the Fischer imaging system can be expected to be 20 to 30 percent higher than on the LORAD biopsy system because of the presence of the stationary, nonreciprocating grid.

Grid Test

As with conventional mammography equipment, acceptance testing should include evaluating the grid for artifacts. For the LORAD biopsy system, which incorporates a reciprocating grid, images should be obtained with the grid moving and stationary, using a 2-cm Lucite block to cover the imaging aperture and using automatic exposure control. The image of the moving grid should show no grid lines when examined with a × 5 magnifying lens. In addition, light streaks or blotches should not be visualized. When imaging the nonmoving, reciprocating LORAD grid or the stationary grid of the Fischer system, grid lines will be visualized; however, they should be regularly spaced and light streaks or artifacts should not be apparent.

ACR Mammography Accreditation Phantom Image

Images of the ACR accreditation phantom can be used for acceptance testing of stereotaxic breast biopsy units. To image the entire phantom, multiple images are necessary. With the usual orientation of the ACR phantom, the fibrils will be imaged at a lower optical density because of the heel effect associated with the prone biopsy units. Therefore, it is necessary to rotate the phantom 180 degrees to accurately test the entire range of artifacts.[13]

Stereotaxic Accuracy

The accuracy of stereotaxic targeting can be tested using the acrylic phantom supplied by the manufacturers; however, homemade or commercial gelatin phantoms provide more realistic evaluations. When performing stereotaxic accuracy tests, it is important to position some targets or artifacts at the corners of the imaging aperture to evaluate the amount of error introduced when a breast lesion cannot be perfectly centered in the biopsy window. This approach is particularly important for testing of digital cameras where CCD defects, pixel dropouts, fiber optic distortions, or inaccurate correction algorithms for fiberoptic distortions will become apparent, resulting in reduced stereotaxic localization accuracy.

When purchasing stereotaxic breast biopsy systems, it is important that the radiologist or hospital administrator ask a physicist with special training in mammography equipment testing to perform the acceptance tests. These evaluations should be thoroughly completed before the equipment is paid for. Because under the requirements of the Mammography Quality Standards Act (MQSA) government agencies may soon mandate periodic testing, it is important that radiologists become familiar with the procedures needed to test prone stereotaxic equipment and the differences in manufacturing designs.

REFERENCES

1. Bolmgren J, Jacobson B, Nordenstrom B. Stereotaxic instrument for needle biopsy of the breast. Am J Roentgenol 1977; 129:121–125.

2. Kaye MD, Vicinanza-Adami CA, Sullivan ML. Mammographic findings after stereotaxic biopsy of the breast performed with large-core needles. Radiology 1994; 192:149–151.

3. Fajardo LL, Davis JR. Mammography-guided fine needle aspiration cytology of nonpalpable breast lesions: prospective comparison with surgical biopsy results. Am J Roentgenol 1990; 155:977–981.

4. Fajardo LL, Jackson VP, Hunter TB. Interventional procedures in diseases of the breast: needle biopsy, pneumocystography, and galactography. Am J Roentgenol 1992; 158:1231–1238.

5. Parker SH, Lovin JD, Jobe WE, et al. Nonpalpable breast lesions: stereotactic automated large-core biopsies. Radiology 1991; 180:403–407.

6. Elvercrog EL, Lechner MC, Nelson MT. Nonpalpable breast lesions: correlation of stereotaxic large-core needle biopsy and surgical biopsy results. Radiology 1993; 188:453–455.

7. Roehrig H, Fajardo LL, Yu T. Digital x-ray cameras for real time stereotactic breast needle biopsy. Proc SPIE 1993; 1896:213–224.

8. Dershaw DD, Fleischman RC, Liberman L, et al. An evaluation of digital mammography by phantom testing and clinical utilization in breast localization procedures. Am J Roentgenol 1993; 161:559–562.

9. Roehrig H, Fajardo LL, Yu T, Schempp WS. Signal, noise, and detective quantum efficiency in CCD based x-ray imaging systems for use in mammography. Proc SPIE 1993; 2163:320–332.

10. Hendrick RE, Parker SH. Stereotaxic imaging. In: Haus AG, Yaffe MJ (eds). A Categorical Course in Physics: Technical Aspects of Breast Imaging. RSNA, Oakbrook, IL, 1993; 233–243.

11. Fajardo LL, Westerman BR. Choosing mammography equipment: technical requirements and practical considerations for the radiologist. Appl Radiol 1990; 19:12–15.

12. Hendrick RE. ACR Mammography Quality Control Manual for Medical Physicist 1992.

13. Kimme-Smith C, Solberg T. Acceptance testing prone stereotactic breast biopsy units. Med Phys 1994; 21:1197–1201.

6

CORE BIOPSY:
GUNS AND NEEDLES

W. Phil Evans

The development of stereotaxic x-ray devices and high resolution ultrasound probes has enabled physicians with experience in breast imaging to guide needles accurately into impalpable breast lesions. Initially coupled with fine needle aspiration (FNA) cytology using 20- to 25-gauge needles, these procedures have demonstrated promising results in the percutaneous cytologic diagnosis of malignant lesions.[1–3] As the limitations of FNA were described, however, enthusiasm diminished. Drawbacks included a paucity of well-trained cytopathologists in the United States, the need for histologic confirmation of malignant aspirates, the high percentage of insufficient samples, and the inability to make a specific benign diagnosis or differentiate in situ from invasive carcinoma.[4]

Removing a cylindrical sample, or core, of tissue with a cutting needle (TruCut) has been used for many years in the diagnosis of palpable breast masses. This technique overcomes the disadvantages of FNA, as many well-trained histopathologists are available, histology is the standard for determining malignancy, insufficient samples are few, and invasive carcinoma can be differentiated from in situ disease. With the development of the automated biopsy gun and its adaptation for stereotactic and sonographic guidance, accurate histologic diagnosis of impalpable breast lesions without surgical biopsy has become a reality.[5–12]

CORE BIOPSY NEEDLES

For core biopsy a specially adapted cutting needle that fits into an automated spring-loaded biopsy gun is used (Fig. 6-1). Needles of various gauges (14 through 20) are commercially available, but the 14-gauge needle gives the most accurate results[13] (Fig. 6-2). It provides a larger volume of tissue, enabling the pathologist to render a more specific histologic diagnosis, yet has a minimal complication rate.

The standard 14-gauge needle used for core biopsy achieves tissue removal in the following manner. The needle assembly is made of stainless steel and consists of an inner tissue sampling needle and outer cutting needle (Fig. 6-3). A 17-mm tissue slot is located 4 mm from the end of the inner needle (Fig. 6-4). The outer needle covers the inner needle in the prebiopsy position. The needle assembly is positioned by stereotaxic or ultrasound guidance with the tip adjacent to the breast lesion.

To perform the biopsy, the inner needle is advanced forward, moving the tissue slot within the lesion (Fig. 6-5). The tip of the inner needle has a downward bevel, which causes it to "dive" slightly during advancement. This downward deflection theoretically allows a relatively larger sample of tissue to be obtained than if the needle advanced directly through the lesion (Fig. 6-6). When advancement of the inner needle is complete and the lesion is within the tissue

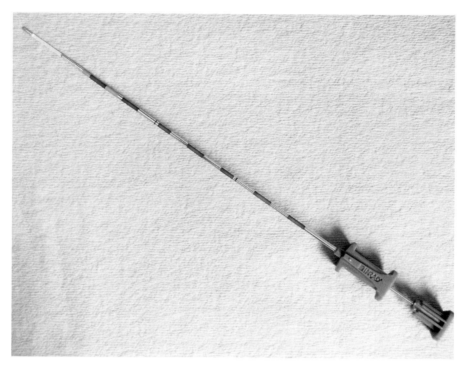

Fig. 6-1. A 14-gauge core biopsy needle adapted for use with an automated biopsy gun (Bard Biopty, Bard Radiology, Covington, Georgia).

slot, the outer needle slides over the inner needle, cutting a tissue sample and securing it in the slot. With an automated biopsy gun, this sequence of events occurs in a split second and is not visible, except for the excursion of the entire needle.

Core biopsy needles are manufactured in several lengths. Generally the longer needles (16 cm) are used with stereotaxic procedures to allow sufficient needle length for placement through two needle guides. The shorter needles (10 cm) are used with ultrasound techniques, as a needle guide is not necessary (Fig. 6-7).

AUTOMATED BIOPSY GUNS

The automated biopsy gun is a small, spring-powered, hand-held medical device. It contains two sets of springs, which rapidly move the two sections of the core biopsy needle, a mechanism for cocking the gun, a safety device, and a trigger. Lindgren,[14] a Swedish radiologist, developed and described its use in 1982. American urologists quickly recognized the

gun's value and began using it for ultrasound-guided transrectal prostate biopsies. While assisting their urology associates, American radiologists began to appreciate the advantages of Lindgren's device. Tissue removal was accomplished in less than a second with excellent quality and little morbidity.

Today, reusable and disposable biopsy guns are commercially available, and both have spring-powered, needle-advancing devices (Figs. 6-8 and 6-9). With the disposable guns, the needle and gun assembly are manufactured as a single unit. The device is used to biopsy one lesion and then discarded. Replacing the disposable needle in a reusable gun after biopsy allows another use. Disposable guns initially were touted to offer less chance of infection than reusable ones, but the incidence of infection is rare regardless of the gun used. Disposable guns cost from $30 to $50 each and reusable ones from $800 to $2,000. If the number of core biopsies per year in a facility is substantial (more than 100), then a reusable gun is clearly more cost effective. Most reusable biopsy guns are less than 15 cm long and easily held in the palm of the hand (Fig. 6-10).

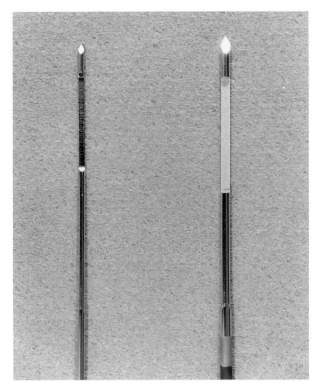

Fig. 6-2. Comparison of 18-gauge (*left*) and 14-gauge (*right*) core biopsy needles. The 14-gauge needle removes twice as much tissue as the 18-gauge needle.

Operating the cocking device compresses the two sets of springs within the gun, one forward and one rearward. When the trigger is depressed, the rear set of springs moves the inner needle forward. With the inner needle in its forward position, tissue enters the slot. During the motion of the rear springs, the forward springs are set in motion, driving the outer cutting needle ahead. A "core" tissue sample is cut and remains in the inner needle slot covered by the outer needle.

Core biopsy with an automated reusable gun is performed as follows. All units have a "door" on top that opens and allows insertion of the biopsy needle into a spring-powered, needle-advancing device (Fig. 6-11). Once the needle is properly positioned in the needle holder, the door is closed. The gun is then "cocked" into the prefire position. When the needle has been positioned adjacent to the lesion to be biopsied, the "safety" is released and the trigger depressed, "firing" the gun, and advancing the needle through the lesion as described previously. The gun and needle are removed from the patient and the tissue sample exposed. Disassembly of the needle and gun is required to extract the tissue sample in the older guns. Newer guns have a two-step cocking procedure that allows removal of the core without removing the needle from the gun. The first cock exposes the tissue slot by retracting the outer needle, and the tissue can be gently removed with a scalpel blade or 18-gauge needle, with or without a saline flush. The second cock retracts the inner needle into the prebiopsy position.

The "throw" of the biopsy gun refers to the distance the needle must travel to obtain a core of tissue. Some guns allow the operator to vary the length of the throw, whereas others are designed for a single throw. The "short throw" (1.0 to 1.5 cm) is not recommended for breast biopsies because of poor tissue samples. The "long throw" (2.1 to 2.5 cm) is preferred in most situations. The maximum dimensions of a tissue core with a long-throw gun and 14-gauge needle are approximately $1 \times 1 \times 17$ mm.

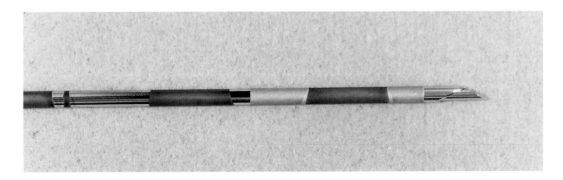

Fig. 6-3. Close-up side view of 14-gauge needle with outer cutting needle covering tissue slot of the inner needle.

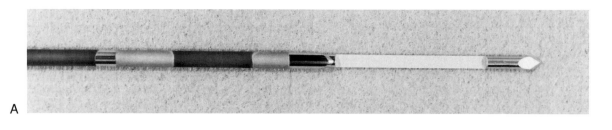

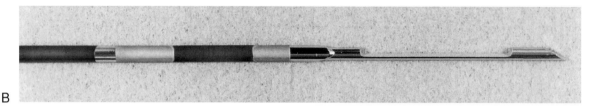

Fig. 6-4. The outer needle has been retracted exposing the 17-mm tissue slot of the 14-gauge needle from the top **(A)** and the side **(B)**. The distance between the tip of the needle and the slot is 4 mm.

When the biopsy gun is fired, the movement of the springs causes a "snapping" sound similar to that of a staple gun. The sound should be demonstrated to the patient before the biopsy to prevent a startled response.

The guns may be cleaned according to manufacturer's recommendations with a 10 percent bleach and water solution, then rinsed with water and air dried. Sterilization of the gun between biopsies is not necessary.

TISSUE CORE SAMPLING

Number

The number of cores needed for biopsy of a lesion is an issue discussed by several investigators.[10,11,15–19] Early reports described authors following specific protocols, removing five cores from each lesion regardless of a lesion's mammographic characteristics. Although five cores are usually the minimum number obtained, the amount removed should be related to the information needed in a particular clinical situation.

Biopsy of most masses generally requires five cores for a specific histologic diagnosis. Visual inspection of the tissue removed is important. Cores of predominantly fatty tissue usually do not yield significant histologic diagnoses. Firm white or gray tissue that sinks in the formalin or saline typically provides satisfactory results.

Lesions manifested solely by microcalcifications (unless the calcifications are relatively large) are generally not visible sonographically and must be sampled stereotaxically. Our approach has been to designate five targets, remove the tissue, and radiograph the specimens. If representative calcifications are present, then the procedure is completed. If calcifications are not seen in the specimen radiograph, however, then five additional targets are selected, and more tissue is removed and radiographed. This procedure can be repeated several times, but we usually stop after 15 to 20 cores (Fig. 6-12). After many cores are selected from one area, specimens may become quite hemorrhagic unless a secondary site has been targeted. Other operators report taking 40 to 50 cores from one area without significant complication (Fred Burbank, M.D., personal communication, 1994).

Specimen Radiography

With microcalcifications, the first goal is to remove a portion of the lesion (calcium), and specimen radiography is essential. The chance of making a specific histologic diagnosis improves significantly if calcification is identified radiographically in the specimens.[16] Specimen radiography is performed with all lesions containing calcium. A glass slide with a metal marker (X-spot) positioned at one end is placed on a cotton 4 × 4 pad. After each biopsy pass, the core of tissue is removed from the needle, delicately placed

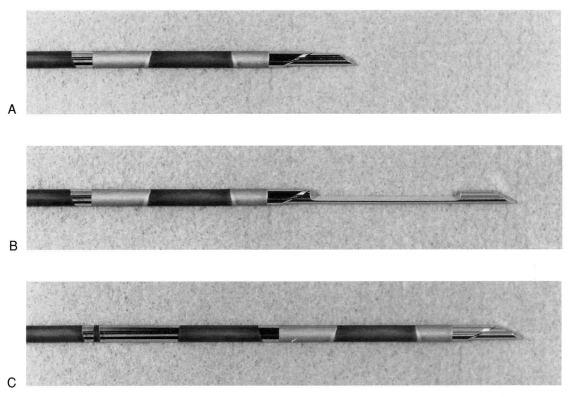

Fig. 6-5. (A) A 14-gauge core needle in prebiopsy position. **(B)** The inner needle has advanced 2.3 cm to uncover the tissue slot. **(C)** The outer needle advances covering the tissue slot. When used with the automated biopsy gun, this movement occurs in a split second.

on the glass slide, and moistened with normal saline. The first core is placed adjacent to the metal marker, with subsequent cores adjacent to the last. After five cores, the 4 × 4 pad and slide are transported for magnification radiography, which can be performed with a standard x-ray unit or dedicated specimen x-ray device (Faxitron). Before filming, tilting the slide will remove the excess saline, allowing it to be absorbed by the 4 × 4 pad. The pad is then discarded, and the specimens on the slide radiographed.

The usual technique factors for magnification specimen radiography are 23 kVp and 20 mAs, but these may vary depending on the film-screen combination. After the film exposure, the cores are moistened again with saline. The metal marker has two purposes. First, if too much magnification is used, there will be geometric distortion and the marker's margins will be blurred on the specimen radiograph. Any chance of imaging calcification will be lost. This distortion is difficult to detect in the specimens alone, but the marker makes recognition simpler. Second, the marker provides a reference point for identifying the specimens. If only two of five specimens contain calcium, these two can be easily identified and sent in a separate container to pathology marked as the calcium-containing cores.

The surrounding tissue that does not contain calcium is also important. In 5 to 24 percent of surgical biopsies for calcifications where malignancy is found, the calcifications are related to a benign process,[20–23] and the malignancy, usually low-grade duct carcinoma in situ, resides in the surrounding tissue. Therefore, with calcifications, removal of adjacent tissue as well as calcium would seem prudent.

Special Situations

In some special clinical situations, one may obtain only a few cores. For example if carcinoma is strongly suspected because of mammographic findings, then one to two cores may be removed and analyzed by frozen section histologic examination. If malig-

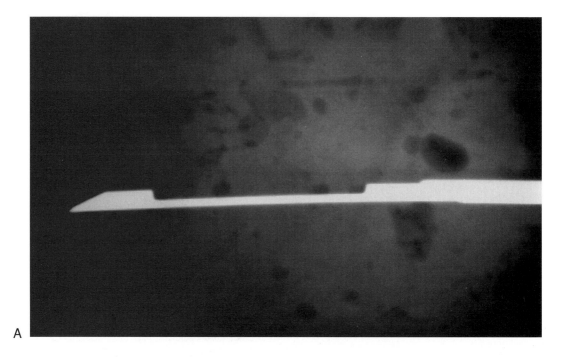

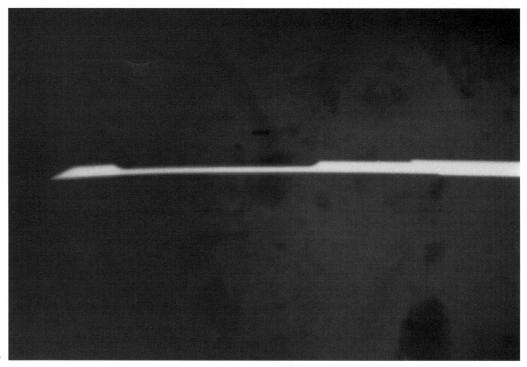

Fig. 6-6. Because of the downward bevel on the tip of the inner needle, its course through the tissue (chicken breast phantom) takes a slightly inferior course, which is greater with the 14-gauge needle **(A)** than with the 18-gauge needle **(B)**.

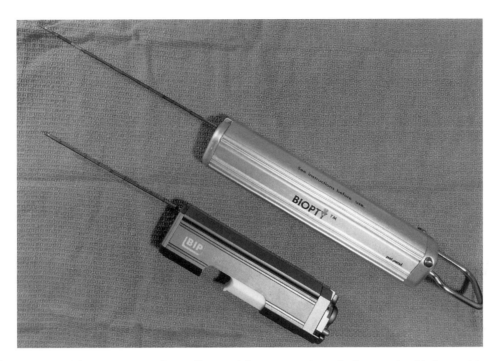

Fig. 6-7. Automated biopsy guns with needles used for stereotaxic and ultrasound-guided core biopsy. The shorter 10-cm needles are used with ultrasound and the longer 16-cm needles are used with stereotaxic biopsy.

nancy can be unequivocally confirmed, the hypothetical risk of tumor seeding through hemorrhage and ecchymosis is minimized with only one or two needle passes. This approach also may be used when a large, locally advanced carcinoma is present, and chemotherapy is likely to be the initial treatment. Three cores of tissue can be removed—one used for histologic diagnosis and estrogen and progesterone receptor immunoassay (ERICA and PRICA) and two for flow cytometry. In this manner appropriate information for treating the patient is obtained without surgical biopsy.

Tissue used for frozen section examination or flow cytometry should not be placed into formalin. To transport the tissue to pathology for freezing, an inverted empty formalin jar may be used. The tissue is positioned in the lid, moistened with normal saline, and the bottom of the jar is screwed into the lid. The inverted position of the jar is maintained throughout transport.

Under all other circumstances, frozen section examination is not recommended for core biopsied tissue, as superior histologic detail is present with permanent sections. This is especially important with

microcalcifications because of possible tissue loss in the microtome with freezing.

THE STEREOTAXIC TECHNIQUE: TARGETING THE LESION

Procedure

The patient's mammogram is reviewed to determine the best approach to the lesion, which in most cases is the skin surface closest to the lesion. Stereotaxically and sonographically guided core biopsies are described in detail in Chapters 9 and 10, but are briefly reviewed here. For stereotaxic biopsies, the breast is compressed within the stereotaxic unit, and a scout image produced with the lesion visible in the 5×5 cm window of the compression device (Fig. 6-13). The skin is prepped with povidone-iodine. Stereo images are obtained with the tube shifted first 15 degrees to the right and then 15 degrees to the left. Using a computerized calculation, the x, y, and z coordinates of a specific target within the lesion (usually the center) are calculated and relayed to the

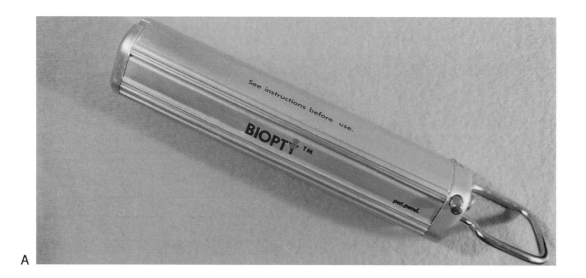

A

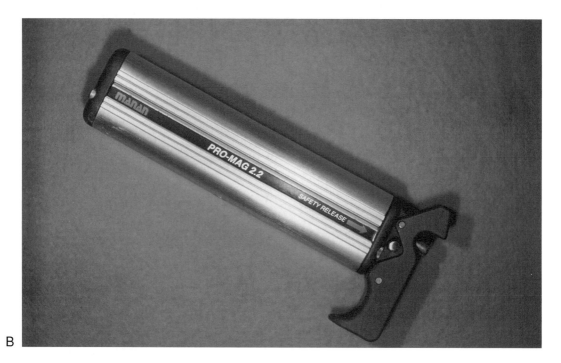

B

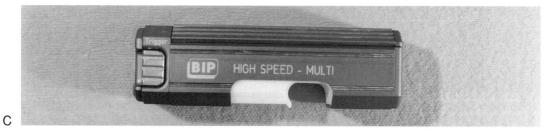

C

Fig. 6-8. Automated biopsy guns. **(A)** Bard Biopty, Bard Radiology, Covington, Georgia. **(B)** Manan Pro-Mag 2.2, Manan Scientific Products, Northbrook, Illinois. **(C)** BIP High Speed Multi, Biopsy-Instruments and Products, Niagara Falls, New York.

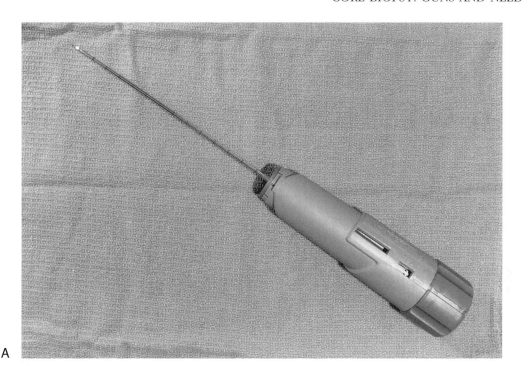

A

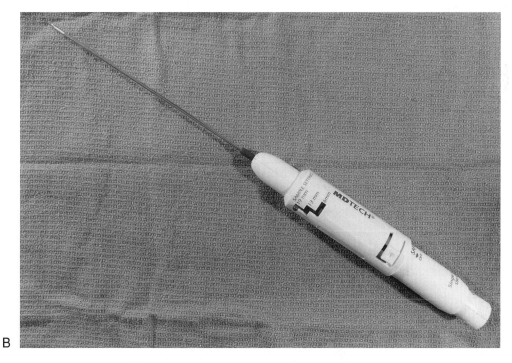

B

Fig. 6-9. Disposable automated biopsy guns. The needle and gun assembly are a single unit and can be discarded after use. **(A)** Bard Monopty, Bard Radiology, Covington, Georgia. **(B)** MD Tech, Gainesville, Florida.

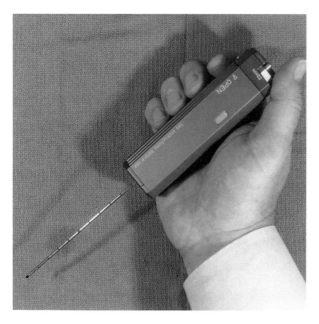

Fig. 6-10. Position for holding the automated biopsy gun for an ultrasound-guided core needle biopsy.

automated biopsy gun and needle holder assembly. The gun and needle holder assembly are positioned with respect to the x and y coordinates. The patient is given local anesthesia (1 percent lidocaine with epinephrine) and a small skin puncture made with a No. 11 blade scalpel over the projected biopsy site. This site can be determined by advancing the needle to the skin and indenting it. Using the z coordinate, the needle is advanced through the skin puncture to the center of the lesion. Stereo images are obtained to confirm placement of the needle within the center of the target.

Before the biopsy gun is fired, the needle is retracted to ensure placement of the inner needle's tissue slot within the center of the lesion. The distance the needle should be retracted depends not only on the size of the lesion and its mobility (Fig. 6-14), but also on the needle gauge and the throw of the gun (Table 6-1). With a 1-cm minimally mobile lesion, 14-gauge needle, and long-throw (2.3 cm) gun, one should retract the needle 0.5 cm. If other factors are unchanged, the needle should be retracted a greater distance with a smaller lesion and a lesser distance with a larger lesion.

After the first firing, stereo views are obtained to document the needle traversing the lesion. The needle is removed and the tissue core placed in a 10 percent formalin solution (Fig. 6-15). Additional cores (usually a total of 5 to 20) are obtained by simply retargeting various areas within the lesion. It generally is not necessary to make a separate puncture for each pass, as the skin nick can be moved without displacing the target within the breast. Core samples may be used to determine estrogen and progesterone receptor status and for flow cytometry studies if indicated.[24]

Each time the needle is removed from the breast, firm pressure is applied to the biopsy site. After the last core is removed, pressure is held for approximately 5 minutes or until bleeding has ceased. An ice pack also may be helpful to minimize bruising.

Digital mammography greatly improves the stereotaxic biopsy procedure, as images may be viewed in a few seconds rather than the several minutes required with standard processing. The rapid image acquisition allows precise prefire needle placement so that highly accurate biopsies can be performed (see Ch. 5). Most stereotaxic biopsies

Table 6-1. Prefire Distance (mm) from Tip of Needle to Center of 1-cm Lesion

	Monopty[a]		Biopty[a]	
Gauge	Short Throw	Long Throw	Short Throw	Long Throw
20	3.5	9.5	-0.9	10.6
18	2.3	8.3	2.1	9.4
16	1.1	7.1	-3.4	8.1
14	-0.5	5.5	-6.0	5.5

[a]Bard Radiology, Covington, Georgia.
Note: Negative number indicates need to place tip of needle partially into lesion.

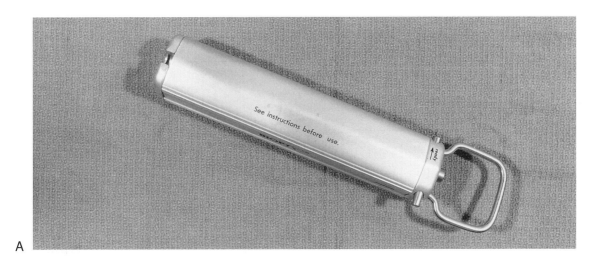

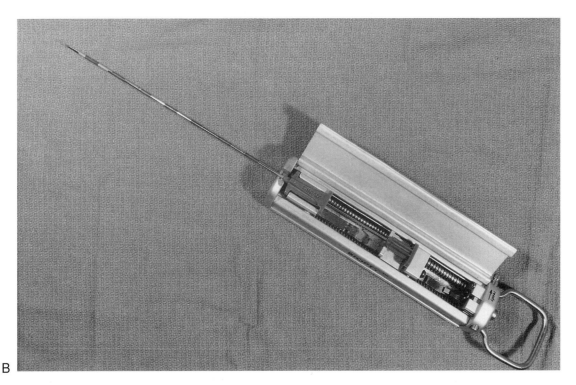

Fig. 6-11. (A) Automated biopsy gun viewed from above with needle "door" closed. **(B)** The needle door is open and a 14-gauge core biopsy needle inserted. Note the uncoiled position of the two sets of springs. *(Figure continues.)*

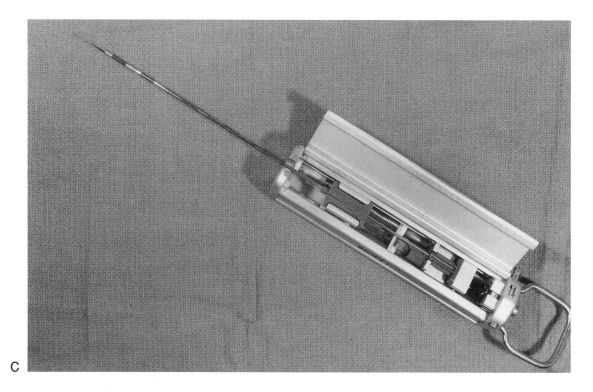

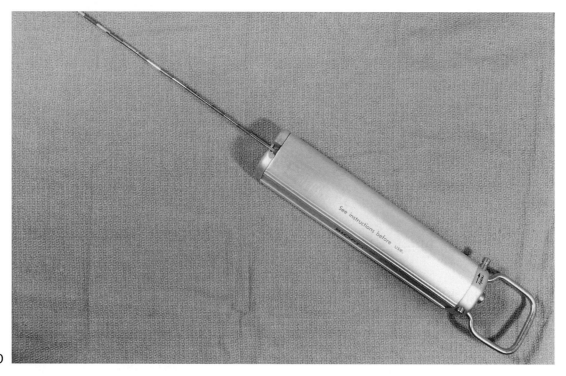

Fig. 6-11. *(Continued).* **(C)** The gun has been cocked, and the door has been left open to demonstrate the coiled position of both sets of springs. **(D)** The door has been closed, and the gun is ready for firing.

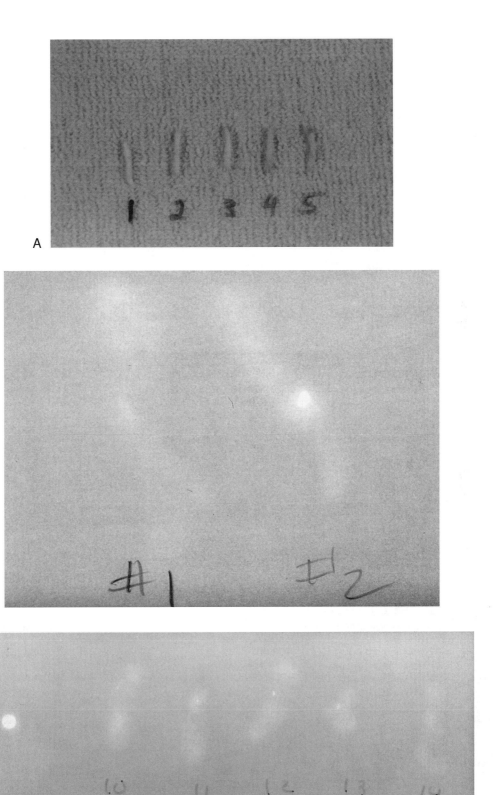

Fig. 6-12. (A) Cores of tissue placed on a glass slide. **(B)** Specimen removed during core biopsy. A large calcification is seen in the second core. **(C)** Specimen radiograph demonstrating removal of calcium in cores 10, 11, 12, and 13. No calcium is present in core 14 or the first 9 cores (not shown).

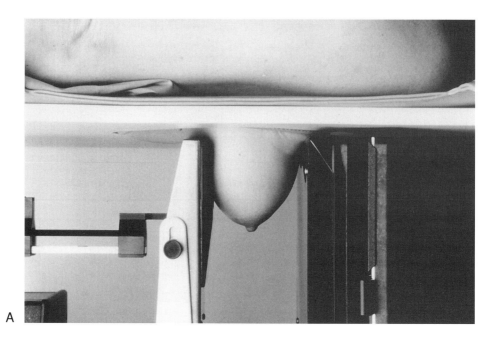

A

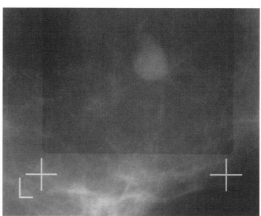

B

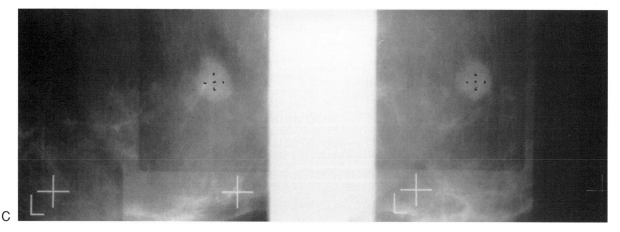

C

Fig. 6-13. (A) The breast is compressed in the stereotaxic unit. **(B)** A scout image of the lesion within the 5 × 5 cm window of the compression device. **(C)** Stereo images with five identical targets marked on each image. *(Figure continues.)*

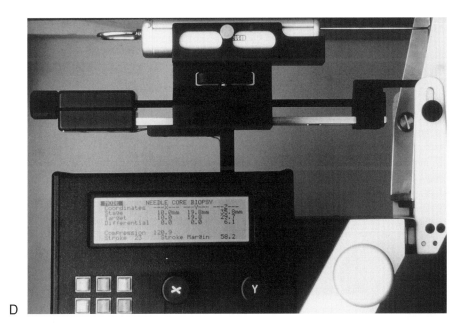

D

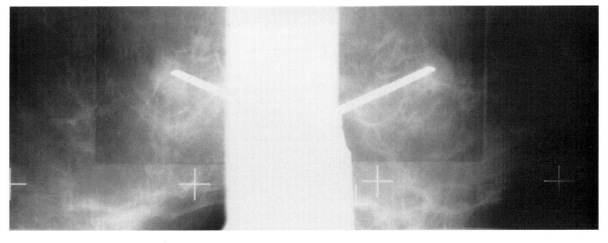

E

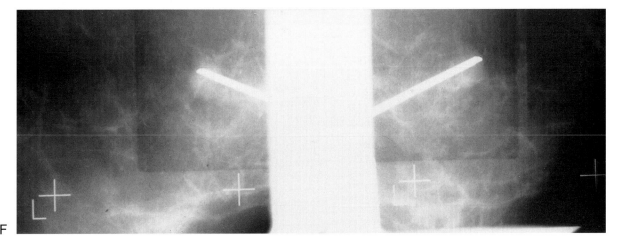

F

Fig. 6-13. *(Continued).* **(D)** The needle is in position to enter the breast. **(E)** Prefire stereo images with the needle in the center of the lesion. **(F)** Postfire images with the needle through the lesion.

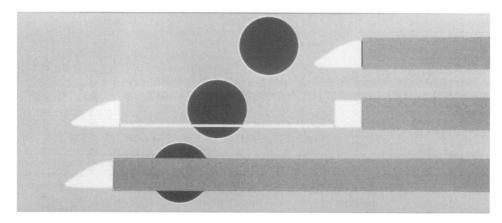

Fig. 6-14. Core needle biopsy, side view. The needle (*upper diagram*) has been retracted from its position in the prefire images in order for the lesion to be within the center of the inner needle tissue slot when it is fired (*middle diagram*). The outer needle moves forward (*lower diagram*), removing a section of the lesion. (Courtesy of Richard Bird, LORAD Corp., Danbury, Connecticut.)

require 45 to 50 minutes from the time the patient enters the room until completion. Digital processing reduces average procedure time 25 to 50 per-cent. Image quality is quite sufficient, and lesion visualization can be improved by varying the contrast, brightness, and magnification (Fig. 6-16).

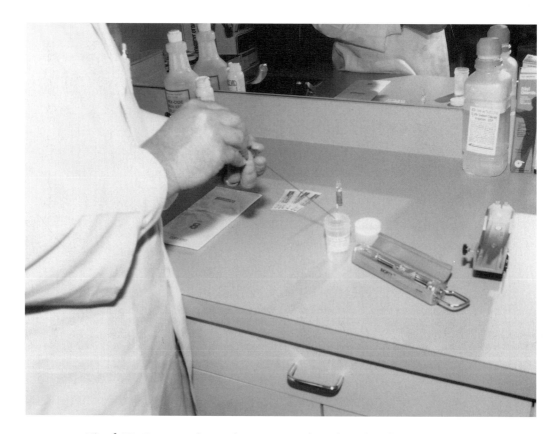

Fig. 6-15. Operator placing the tissue sample in formalin after core biopsy.

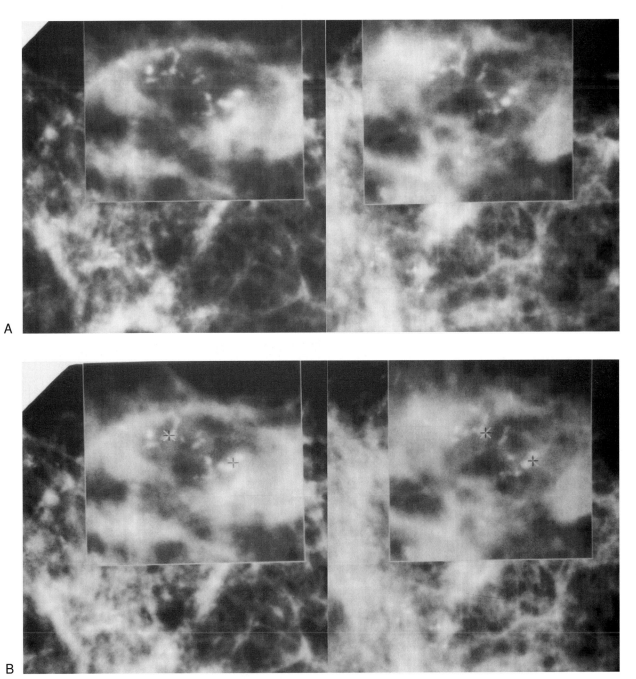

A

B

Fig. 6-16. Digital stereo images of microcalcifications. **(A)** The visualization of the calcifications in the region of interest is improved by magnification and contrast enhancement. **(B)** Two specific calcifications have been targeted electronically for core biopsy. (*Figure continues.*)

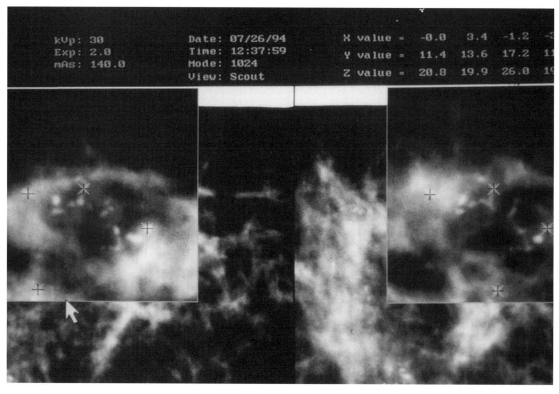

kVp: 30	Date: 07/26/94	X value = -0.0 3.4 -1.2 -3
Exp: 2.0	Time: 12:37:59	Y value = 11.4 13.6 17.2 11
mAs: 140.0	Mode: 1024	Z value = 20.8 19.9 26.0 19
	View: Scout	

C

Fig. 6-16. (*Continued*). (**C**) Targeting with multitarget function. The four precise targets have unique x, y, and z coordinates.

Masses

Targeting a spherical or ovoid mass using stereotaxic technique is a relatively simple procedure. After obtaining stereo images of the mass, targets are marked first at the center and then at the 12, 3, 6, and 9 o'clock positions of the lesion on each image. This step can be accomplished electronically with digital mammography units using a computer track ball (Fig. 6-17) or manually with film-screen units using a film illuminator and a pencil (Fig. 6-13). The operator should carefully mark the same point on the mass on each image to allow accurate calculation of the target's x, y, and z coordinates.

To assist in targeting, most commercially available digital stereotaxic units have "multipass" and "multitarget" capability. With the multipass function, the lesion's center target is marked on both stereo images, and the x, y, and z coordinates are calculated. The remaining targets can now be marked on just one of the digital stereo images to complete targeting because only one view is necessary to determine a lesion's x and y coordinates, whereas two views are needed to calculate the z coordinate (depth). The z coordinate calculated for the center lesion is used for all other targets. The multipass function is used to biopsy masses since the z coordinate is the same for each target. The multitarget function is used to biopsy microcalcifications because unique x, y, and z coordinates are needed for each target (Fig. 6-16C).

The most common reason for a needle biopsy "miss" is movement of the breast or lesion within the breast. Use of too much local anesthetic can obscure the target or move it significantly (Fig. 6-18). Moreover, some lesions, usually fibroadenomas, are quite firm and can be displaced by the needle. Only with precisely positioned prefire images and confirming postfire images can one be reasonably certain that the lesion has been biopsied.

Microcalcifications

Microcalcifications may have a spherical (clustered), linear, segmental, or irregular distribution. In some instances, the most suspicious calcifications may be

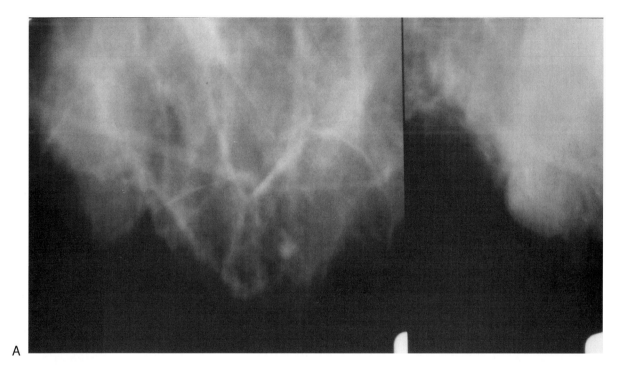

A

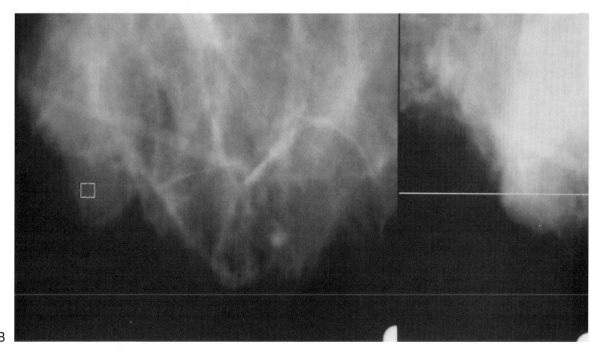

B

Fig. 6-17. Targeting with multipass function. **(A)** Digital stereo images of a mass. **(B–D)** The center of the lesion is targeted on each image. (*Figure continues.*)

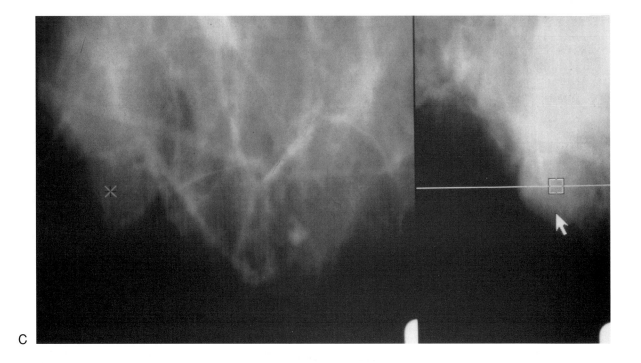

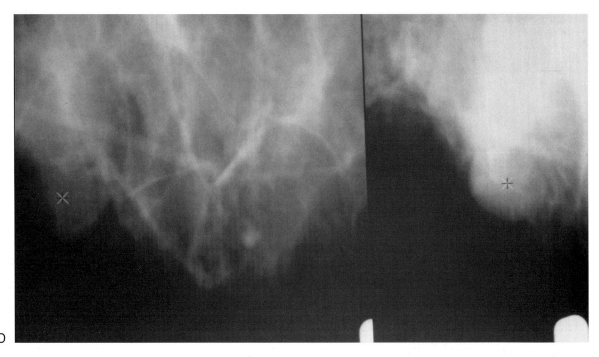

Fig. 6-17. (*Figure continues*).

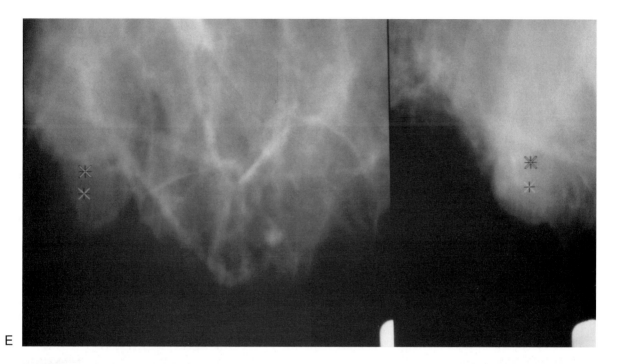

E

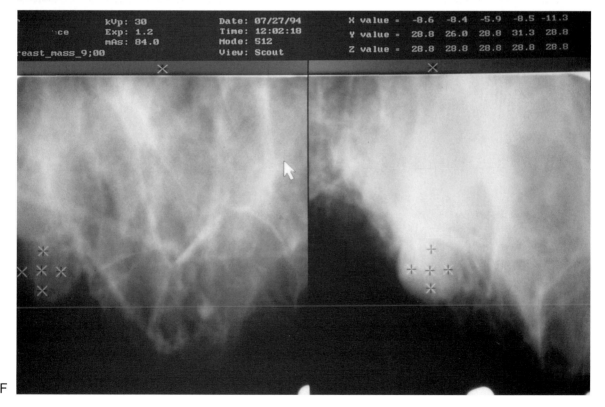

F

Fig. 6-17. *(Continued).* **(E)** Subsequent targets need be marked only on the left image. **(F)** The x and y coordinates are unique for each target, but the z coordinate is the same.

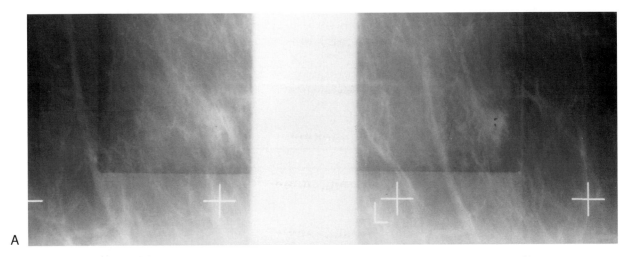

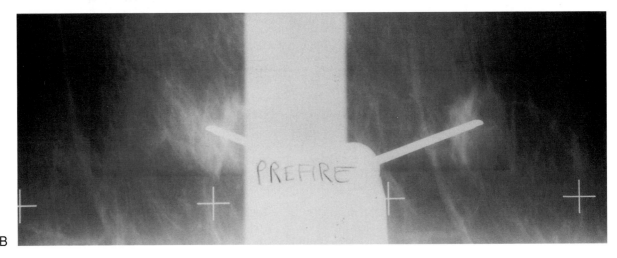

Fig. 6-18. (A) Prefire images of small invasive carcinoma. **(B)** Use of excessive local anesthetic obscures the lesion.

erratically disbursed throughout the lesion. Therefore, the areas to be biopsied and the number of cores needed must be selected carefully.

A tightly packed sphere or cluster of relatively large pleomorphic microcalcifications commonly seen with localized comedocarcinoma is usually the easiest of this group to target (Fig. 6-19). This lesion may be targeted in a manner similar to a mass; however, only by targeting the same calcification on each stereo image will accurate needle placement be achieved (Fig. 6-16).

Microcalcifications distributed in a linear, segmental, or irregular manner are more difficult to biopsy, as they present a smaller target over a larger area (Fig. 6-20). With any one of the these patterns, the center of the most morphologically suspicious calcifications—where several flecks of calcium are clustered closely together—provide the best target.

Again the same calcification on each stereo image must be identified and meticulously targeted. Even if targeting is inaccurate by only 1 mm in the x or y axis, there is a significant chance that calcium will not be removed. Frequently with large areas of calcification, the best target is the lesion's periphery where the most diagnostic histologic information may be found (Fig. 6-21).

THE ULTRASOUND TECHNIQUE: TARGETING THE LESION

Procedure

Sonographically guided core biopsy is technically more difficult to perform than stereotaxically guided biopsy. Targeting begins with rescanning the patient

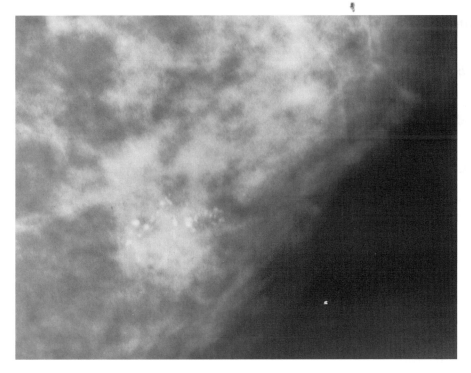

Fig. 6-19. A tightly grouped cluster of microcalcifications related to comedo-type duct carcinoma in situ. This distribution of calcifications is relatively easy to target.

and marking the lesion on the skin to determine the best approach. The needle should be directed as near parallel to the chest wall as possible. Generally this maneuver can be accomplished by placing the patient in an oblique position and following the curve of the chest wall with the needle entry site (Figs. 6-22 and 6-23).

The skin is prepped with povidone-iodine. A sterile cover (condom) filled with ultrasound gel is placed over the transducer. Absolute alcohol can be used as the sonographic coupling medium and is applied to the skin with cotton 4 × 4 pads (Fig. 6-24). The lesion is again located. The simplest and most accurate needle path to the lesion is along the long axis of the transducer. Therefore, after local anesthetic, a small skin incision is made at the edge of the transducer, and the needle is advanced obliquely along the transducer's long axis. With lesions deep in the breast near the chest wall, the skin incision must be made at a greater distance from the transducer to maintain needle position parallel to the chest wall.

The needle must be kept within the focal plane of the transducer or it cannot be visualized. This maneuver is the most difficult and critical part of the biopsy.

The operator has one hand on the transducer and guides the needle into position with the other hand. The needle is advanced to the edge of the lesion (Fig. 6-25). An assistant may be needed to fire the gun, although some newer guns are designed so that the operator can both hold and fire the gun with the same hand. After determining that the needle path will not enter the pectoralis muscle or chest wall, the biopsy gun is fired and the lesion sampled. The core specimen is removed, visually evaluated for adequacy, placed in 10 percent formalin, and the procedure repeated.

Usually five cores are satisfactory for histologic evaluation of masses. As with the stereotactic technique, it is important to sample different areas within the lesion on each needle pass. The center, 12 o'clock, and 6 o'clock targets are obtained initially, and then by slightly changing the position of the transducer, the 3 and 9 o'clock targets are sampled. Both prefire and postfire images are made to document needle placement through the lesion.

When the needle is removed from the breast on each pass, pressure is applied to the biopsy site. With ultrasound guided biopsies, it is important to note that the skin nick is *not* where pressure should be applied,

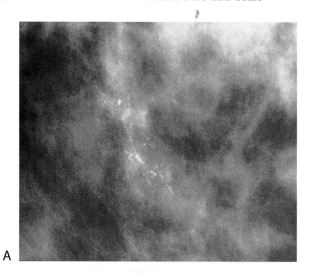

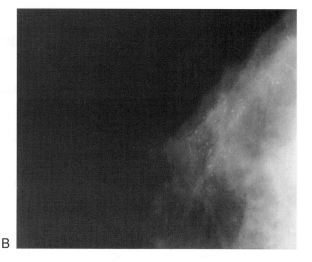

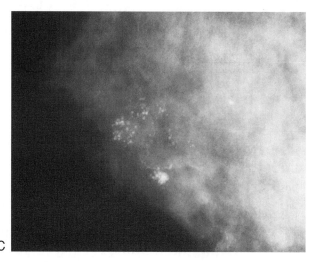

Fig. 6-20. Microcalcifications distributed in **(A)** a linear, **(B)** segmental, and **(C)** irregular pattern. Targeting of these calcifications is relatively more difficult than with a localized cluster.

but rather over the needle track and the lesion several centimeters away. Considerable bleeding around the lesion may occur unless pressure is properly applied and held for approximately 5 minutes or until all bleeding has ceased. An ice pack also may be helpful.

Special Situations

On rare occasions, one may encounter breast tissue so dense that the springs in the automated biopsy gun are not powerful enough to propel the needle through the tissue. In this situation, the inner needle will advance, but the outer needle will not, resulting in an open needle slot in the breast. Some difficulty in removing the

needle from the patient's breast will be encountered. Usually by gently recocking the gun, the inner needle will retract, allowing easier removal.

To remove a core from very dense tissue, it may be necessary to manually move the needle through the lesion making a track. Then the gun may be fired and the needle moved through the lesion successfully.

A coaxial core biopsy system has been developed so that a new track through the tissue need not be made with each needle pass.[25] This device may be helpful in some circumstances, although with most ultrasound-guided biopsies, the initial needle pathway to the lesion can be used easily with each pass.

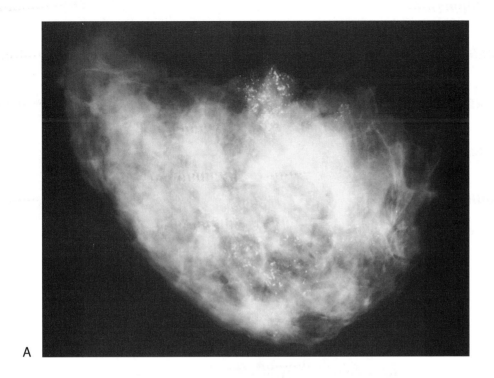

A

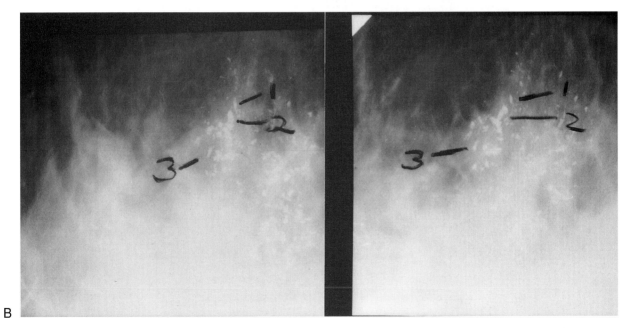

B

Fig. 6-21. (A) Extensive comedocarcinoma involving most of the breast but not producing a definite palpable lesion. Blind core biopsy results were benign. **(B)** Stereo images of calcifications on the posterior margin of the lesion with the same calcification targeted in each view.

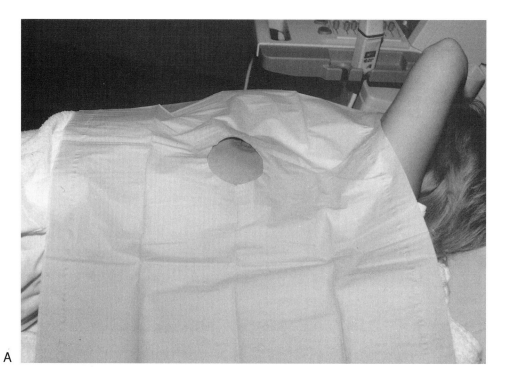

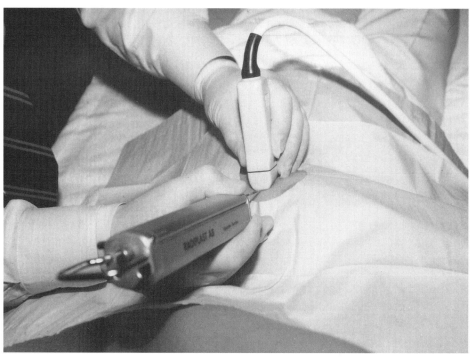

Fig. 6-22. (A) The patient has been placed in the right posterior oblique position for ultrasound guided biopsy of a lesion in the outer portion of the left breast. Her left arm is extended above her head. Use of the drape is optional. Lesions in the medial portion of the breast may be biopsied with the patient in a supine position. **(B)** The transducer is held in one hand and the biopsy gun in the other. The needle path is within the focal plane of the transducer.

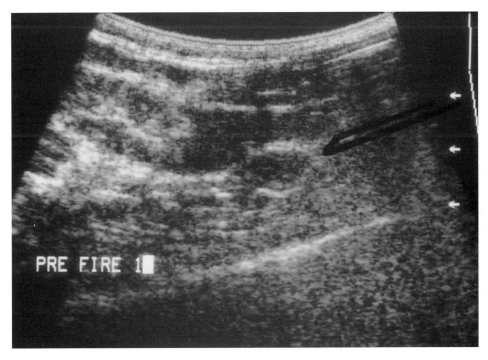

Fig. 6-23. The needle is almost parallel to the chest wall as it approaches the lesion. If the needle were to approach from the opposite direction, it would be almost perpendicular to the chest wall when the gun was fired.

INDICATIONS: BENEFITS AND PITFALLS

With increasing emphasis on outpatient procedures, the surgical treatment of breast cancer is usually a two-stage process: surgical biopsy followed by a definitive procedure, either lumpectomy, with or without axillary dissection, or mastectomy, with or without reconstruction. Core needle biopsy is changing this paradigm and offers clear advantages over surgery in several instances. First, lesions of low-intermediate suspicion, particularly those with a 10 to 30 percent chance of malignancy, are ideal for core needle biopsy. In most cases, the procedure shortens the diagnostic process, achieving a specific benign diagnosis and replacing surgical biopsy. If malignancy is found, a definitive surgical procedure may be performed. Second, lesions with high mammographic suspicion of malignancy in patients who wish to have a mastectomy, with or without reconstruction, rather than lumpectomy can be definitively diagnosed by core biopsy, thereby avoiding surgical biopsy. Finally, patients with lesions characterized by multiple clusters of microcalcifications or multiple masses in different quadrants of the same breast may be excluded from breast conservation if two or more can be proved malignant by core biopsy. The patient can proceed with mastectomy, with or without reconstruction, with no surgical biopsy.

Almost any breast lesion is suitable for core needle biopsy, but in a few instances, it is not helpful. If the histologic diagnosis of a lesion by needle biopsy will not shorten the diagnostic process, if removal of the entire lesion is necessary for accurate diagnosis, or if a lesion cannot be targeted successfully, then core biopsy is not recommended.

Although lesions with a low-intermediate mammographic suspicion of malignancy are well suited for core biopsy, its role with high-suspicion lesions (80 percent or greater chance of malignancy), when breast conservation is the treatment of choice, is controversial. Some surgeons prefer excisional biopsy as the first diagnostic and therapeutic maneuver. They contend that the patient can observe the lumpectomy's cosmetic result before axillary node dissection and radiation therapy. The presence or absence of an extensive intraductal component (EIC) can be determined, and the surgical margins assessed. If the surgical margins are

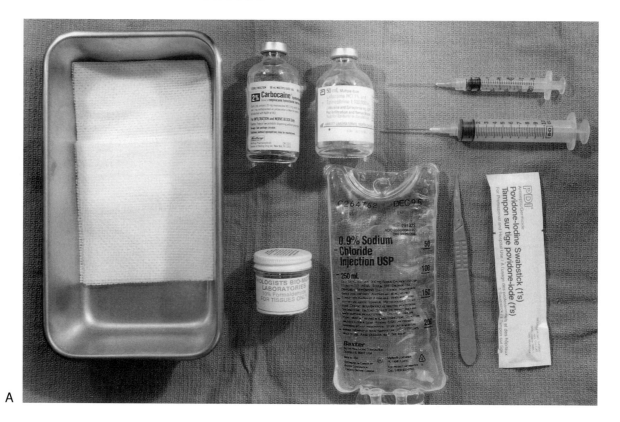

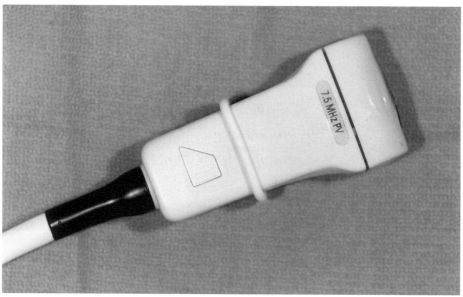

Fig. 6-24. (A) Tray for ultrasound-guided core needle biopsy. Alcohol soaked 4 × 4 pads used to apply the coupling agent, No. 11 scalpel blade, povidone-iodine, 10 cc syringe (18-gauge, 1-in needle) with normal saline to assist in removing the core from the biopsy needle, bottle of 10 percent formalin, and a 3 cc-syringe (25-gauge, 1.5-in needle) for local anesthesia (1 percent lidocaine with epinephrine or 2 percent carbocaine). **(B)** Ultrasound transducer fitted with a condom filled with ultrasound gel.

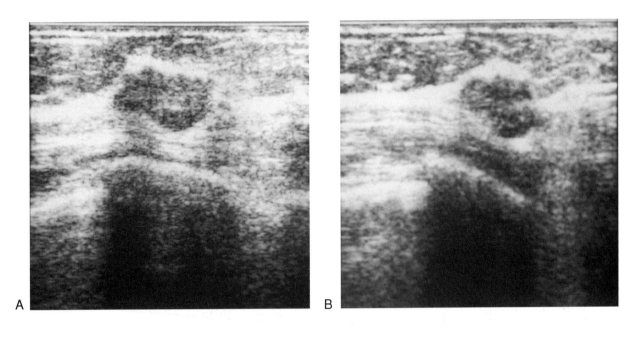

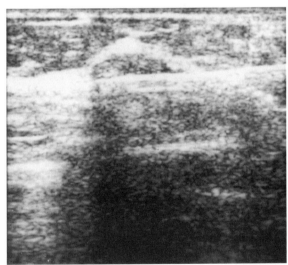

Fig. 6-25. (A) Sonographic image of a 1.3-cm impalpable mass adjacent to the chest wall. **(B)** The 14-gauge needle has been positioned parallel to the chest wall, with the tip abutting to the mass. **(C)** The gun is fired and the needle passes through the lesion. *(Figure continues.)*

not free of tumor, re-excision can be performed before axillary dissection. As many as 76 percent of lumpectomies may require re-excision because of involved margins.[26] In this two-step scenario, core needle biopsy, it is argued, is an added expense.

Other surgeons assert that a presurgical malignant diagnosis permits discussion of treatment options

before surgery and a greater chance of performing a lumpectomy with adequate margins in a single procedure. These differences seem to be related to surgical technique preferences and the volume of breast tissue removed during lumpectomy. Based on experience at Baylor University Medical Center, surgical breast cancer treatment can be successfully performed in most

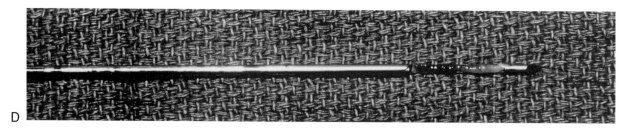

D

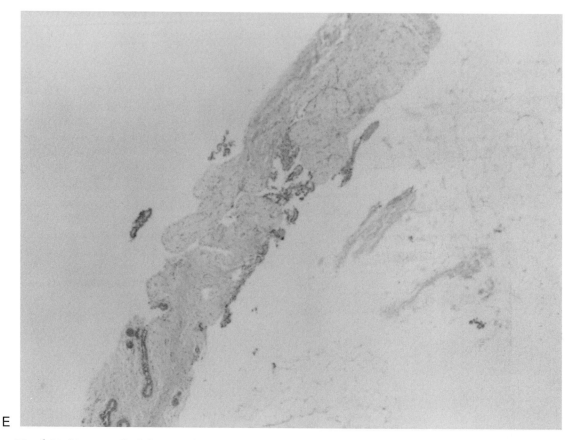

E

Fig. 6-25 *(Continued).* **(D)** Core of tissue removed during needle biopsy. **(E)** Histologic section of tissue core removed during the biopsy demonstrating a fibroadenoma.

cases (89%) after core biopsy for malignancy, with only one surgical procedure (Table 6-2).

The histologic diagnosis of the radial scar or complex sclerosing lesion, even when totally excised, may be a difficult histologic diagnosis (Fig. 6-26). Its assessment, therefore, becomes an even greater (although not impossible) challenge from only core samples. Hence with suspected radial scars, surgical rather than core needle biopsy is advised. Papillary lesions and some forms of sclerosing adenosis also fall into this category.

Although very small lesions can be accurately sampled, large areas of granular microcalcifications may be difficult to target stereotaxically and require surgical biopsy for diagnosis. This lesion may also harbor low-grade duct carcinoma in situ (DCIS) unrelated to the microcalcifications.

Some patients or their lesions may not be technically suited for stereotaxic biopsy. Women who cannot lie prone or undergo extended breast compression are not candidates for the procedure. If a breast lesion is very superficial or the breast compresses to

Table 6-2. Surgical Treatment of Malignant Lesions[a]

Surgical Therapy	Total Number	Number With One Surgical Procedure After Core Biopsy	Number With > 1 Surgical Procedure After Core Biopsy
Mastectomy	95	91	4
Lumpectomy and axillary dissection	63	51	12
Lumpectomy only	13	11	2
Total	171	153 (89%)	18 (11%)

[a]Diagnosed by Core Biopsy at the Susan G. Komen Breast Center, Dallas, Texas, June 1990 to December 1994. Eighty-nine percent had definitive therapy with only one procedure after core biopsy.

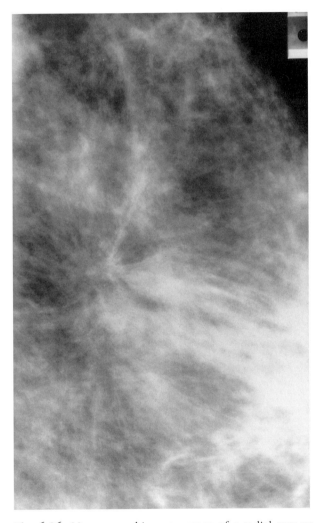

Fig. 6-26. Mammographic appearance of a radial scar or complex sclerosing lesion. Core biopsy of this lesion should be avoided, as removal of the entire lesion is usually necessary for diagnosis. Cores of this lesion may be confused pathologically with low-grade invasive duct carcinoma.

2 cm or less, the biopsy usually cannot be performed. Because of the 2.1 to 2.5 cm throw, the needle tip would need to begin its excursion outside the breast in order for the tissue slot to be properly positioned after firing. Finally, some lesions situated against the chest wall cannot be imaged satisfactorily with the stereotaxic device.

Stereotaxic and ultrasound core breast biopsies are not replacements for an excellent imaging evaluation. The same criteria used in recommending surgical biopsy should be used for core biopsy. Lesions categorized as "probably benign" (i.e., having less than a 2 percent chance of malignancy) usually should undergo periodic mammographic follow-up rather than biopsy. In some circumstances, however, core biopsy of such a lesion may be appropriate because of patient or physician anxiety.[27]

COMPLICATIONS

Complications from core biopsy are rare and include hematoma, infection, and possible tumor seeding. Parker's multicenter study noted six complications (0.2 percent) in 3,765 cases where follow-up was available.[11] Three hematomas required surgical drainage and three infections required drainage and/or antibiotic treatment. Minor bruising around the biopsy site is common but can be minimized by maintaining pressure and using ice when the needle has been removed. Even if a small artery is biopsied, local pressure will usually stop any bleeding. Patients on anticoagulant therapy can be biopsied if the medication is reduced to the lowest acceptable level, and meticulous technique with ice is used in both the prebiopsy and postbiopsy.

Needle tract seeding has been reported in a case of core-biopsied mucinous carcinoma in which the lesion and tract were surgically excised.[28] Malignant cells may be displaced into normal tissue with any needle procedure including FNA and needle localization. Whether these cells are viable or pose any threat to the patient is unknown. Surgical excision of the needle tract when feasible may be an option. Parker et al.[11] reported no cases of needle tract seeding in their series.

SUMMARY

Core needle biopsy using either stereotaxic, x-ray, or ultrasound guidance is a reasonable and accurate alternative to surgical biopsy for diagnosis of most impalpable breast lesions. Meticulous operator technique is essential to provide representative samples of the mammographic abnormality. Performed appropriately, these techniques have great potential for reducing morbidity from surgical breast biopsy and the overall cost of breast cancer diagnosis.

ACKNOWLEDGMENT

Mollie Standish provided invaluable assistance in the preparation of this chapter.

REFERENCES

1. Dowlatshahi K, Gent JH, Schmidt R, et al. Nonpalpable breast tumors: diagnosis with stereotaxic localization and fine-needle aspiration. Radiology 1989; 170:427–433.
2. Ciatto S, Del Turco Mr, Bravetti P. Nonpalpable breast lesion: stereotaxic fine-needle aspiration cytology. Radiology 1989; 173:57–59.
3. Azavedo E, Svane G, Auer G. Stereotaxic fine-needle biopsy in 2,594 mammographically detected non-palpable lesions. Lancet 1989; 1:1033–1036.
4. Jackson VP. The status of mammographically guided fine needle aspiration biopsy of nonpalpable breast lesions. In: Bassett LW (ed). Breast Imaging: Current Status and Future Directions. Radiol Clin North Am 1992; 30:155–166.
5. Parker SH, Lovin JD, Jobe WE, et al. Stereotactic breast biopsy with a biopsy gun. Radiology 1990; 176:741–747.
6. Parker SH, Lovin JD, Jobe WE, et al. Non-palpable breast lesions: stereotactic automated large-core biopsies. Radiology 1991; 180:403–407.
7. Dowlatshahi K, Yaremko ML, Kluskens LF, Jokich PM. Nonpalpable breast lesions: findings of stereotaxic needle-core biopsy and fine-needle aspiration cytology. Radiology 1991; 181:745–750.
8. Dronkers DJ. Stereotaxic core biopsy of breast lesions. Radiology 1992; 183:631–634.
9. Elvecrog EL, Lechner MC, Nelson MT. Non-palpable breast lesions: correlation of stereotaxic large-core needle biopsy and surgical biopsy results. Radiology 1993; 188:453–455.
10. Gisvold JJ, Goellner JR, Grant CS, et al. Breast biopsy: a comparative study of stereotaxically guided core and excisional techniques. Am J Roentgenol 1994; 162:815–820.
11. Parker S, Burbank F, Tabar L, et al. Percutaneous large core breast biopsy: a multi-institutional experience. Radiology 1994; 193:359–364.
12. Parker SH, Jobe WE, Dennis MA, et al. US-guided automated large-core breast biopsy. Radiology 1993; 187:507–511.
13. Chough D, Nath ME, Robinson TM, et al. Automated biopsy needle core biopsies of surgically removed breast specimens. A comparison of core specimens from 14, 16 and 18 gauge. Abstract presented at American Roentgen Ray Society Meeting, New Orleans, 1994.
14. Lindgren PG. Percutaneous needle biopsy: a new technique. Acta Radiol Diagn (Stockh) 1982; 23:653–656.
15. Sullivan DC. Needle core biopsy of mammographic lesions. Am J Roentgenol 1994; 162:601–608.
16. Liberman L, Evans WP, Dershaw DD, et al. Radiography of microcalcifications in stereotaxic mammary core biopsy specimens. Radiology 1994; 190:223–225.
17. Brenner RJ, Bassett LW, Dershaw DD, et al. Percutaneous core biopsy of the breast: a multisite prospective trial. Abstract presented at the Radiological Society of North America 80th Scientific Assembly and General Meeting, Chicago, 1994.
18. Liberman L, Dershaw D, Rosen PP, et al. Stereotaxic 14-gauge breast biopsy: how many core biopsy specimens are needed? Radiology 1994; 192:793–795.
19. Jackman RJ, Nowels KW, Shepard MJ, et al. Stereotaxic large-core needle biopsy of 450 nonpalpable breast lesions with surgical correlation in lesions with cancer or atypical hyperplasia. Radiology 1994; 193:91–95.
20. Murphy WA, DeSchryver-Kesckemeli K. Isolated clustered microcalcifications in the breast: radiologic-pathologic correlation. Radiology 1978; 27:335–341.
21. Roses DR, Harris MN, Gorstein F, Gumport SL: Biopsy for microcalcification detected by mammography. Surgery 1980; 87:248–252.
22. Colbassani HJ, Feller WF, Cigtay OS, Chun B. Mammography and pathologic correlation of microcalcification in disease of the breast. Surg Gynecol Obstet 1982; 155:689–696.

23. Homer MJ, Safaii H, Smith TJ, Marchant DJ. The relationship of mammographic microcalcification to histologic malignancy: radiologic-pathologic correlation. An J Roentgenol 1989; 153:1187–1189.

24. Lovin JD, Sinton EB, Burke BJ, Reddy VV. Stereotaxic core breast biopsy: value in providing tissue for flow cytometric analysis. Am J Roentgenol 1994; 162:609–612.

25. Kaplan SS, Racenstein MJ, Wong WS, et al. US-guided core biopsy of the breast with a coaxial system. Radiology 1995; 194:573–575.

26. Tafra L, Guenther JM, Guiliano AE. Planned segmentectomy: a necessity for breast carcinoma. Arch Surg 1993; 128:1014–1020.

27. Sickles EA, Parker SH. Appropriate role of core breast biopsy in the management of probably benign lesions. Radiology 1993; 188:315.

28. Harter LP, Curtis JS, Ponto G, Craig PH. Malignant seeding of the needle track during stereotaxic core needle breast biopsy. Radiology 1995; 185:713–714.

7 FINE NEEDLE ASPIRATION BIOPSY OF BREAST LESIONS

Etta D. Pisano

Although screening mammography along with breast physical examination has reduced breast cancer mortality, the cost and anxiety associated with screening are increased by the volume of false-positive studies that generate breast biopsies.[1] As has been previously noted, only 10 to 30 percent of lesions that undergo needle localization and open surgical biopsy prove to be malignant.[2] The use of additional procedures, such as short-term mammographic follow-up, can reduce the number of benign lesions that are biopsied.[3,4] In any practice, however, the number of biopsies performed for these lesions is considerable.

Generally speaking, morbidity from open biopsy of nonpalpable lesions is minimal.[5] The financial cost of open surgical biopsy for benign lesions is approximately 32 percent of the total cost of screening.[6] According to Eddy et al.,[7] if screening is performed on women under 50 years old, the total dollars spent for work-up for false-positive mammograms in this age group alone would amount to $40,654,000 in 1984 dollars in the year 2000.[7] Clearly, this expenditure is a significant drain on a burdened health care system. The availability of a less expensive biopsy method might save a large sum of money.

At least partially because of the expense and morbidity of open surgical biopsy, fine needle aspiration biopsy (FNAB) of the breast has been developed. This procedure provides precise percutaneous sampling of both palpable and nonpalpable lesions. Potentially, it can eliminate the need for many costly open surgical procedures, with minimal patient morbidity and without the disfigurement of open biopsy. To perform the procedure successfully, however, some experience with the technique is necessary. High insufficient sampling rates have been reported by those with limited experience. It is also necessary to have a pathologist competent in the interpretation of breast cytology, and such expertise may not be readily available in all practices. Unlike other breast biopsy techniques, FNAB may be performed optimally with both the radiologist and cytologist (or cytopathologist) in the room during the biopsy.

PATIENT SELECTION

A review of the literature reveals that virtually all types of mammographic and palpable lesions have been submitted to FNAB. Unfortunately, no single study has included enough patients of each type to make statistically valid claims about the utility of this tool for each individual type of mammographic finding. In fact, few authors have reported their accuracy data with respect to the type of lesion being sampled.[8–12] Large, multicenter studies are needed to ascertain whether FNAB is better suited for particular types of mammographic lesions.

In general, any mammographically or clinically detected lesion that is accessible to a needle can be subjected to FNAB. Although not strictly contraindicated, patients for whom FNAB might be difficult are those who have known bleeding disorders or are on anticoagulant therapy, are allergic to local anesthesia, have breast implants, or have a psychiatric or neurologic condition that would limit their ability to cooperate during the procedure and give acceptable informed consent.

TECHNIQUE

Equipment

For either sonographically or mammographically guided fine needle aspiration of nonpalpable breast lesions, the following equipment is used: 10-, 20-, or 30-ml plastic syringe with Luer-Lok tip, a cotton swab soaked with alcohol or Betadine solution, 22-, 23-, or 25-gauge disposable needles with transparent plastic hubs, fully frosted glass slides and nonfrosted glass slides, 95 percent alcohol fixative, and 50 percent Ringer's lactate/50 percent alcohol rinse solution, or a balanced salt or Cytolyt rinse solution. A syringe holder, tubing, and local anesthesia are optional. If ultrasound guidance is used, sterile ultrasound gel will be necessary and a sterile transducer drape is optional.

The type of needle used is not that important. It is best to get advice from the local cytopathologist regarding what type of needle he or she prefers. Any of the following brand names can be used (although this list is not exhaustive): Chiba, Franzen, (Manan Medical Products), Northbrook IL; Inrad, Grand Rapids, MI; and BD (Bector-Dickinson), Franklin Lakes, NJ. The needle length depends on the depth of the lesion within the breast. For superficial lesions, 3.8-cm long needles are usually adequate. Longer needles (7 to 9 cm) may be needed for deeper lesions.

Patient Preparation

After explaining the procedure to the patient and obtaining written informed consent, the patient is positioned for placement of the needles. Patient position varies depending on the guidance system used.

For stereotaxic guidance, the patient's breast is placed in the stereotaxic device so that the needles will pass through the smallest amount of breast tissue possible. For most lesions and most machines, the skin surface closest to the lesion can be punctured. For units that do not allow skin entry from the inferior aspect of the breast, the breast should be positioned in a manner that will allow for the shortest practical path to the lesion. For machines with a detachable side arm, the needle path can be directed either perpendicular or parallel to the path of the x-ray beam. For all other machines, the needle path will be parallel to the path of the beam.

The breast should be positioned so that the lesion lies as close as possible to the central x-ray beam. A scout image is obtained to confirm that the lesion is appropriately situated. If the lesion is small or of low contrast and difficult to visualize, a radiographic grid may be used to obtain the scout view. If the lesion position is not optimally seen on this scout view, the breast should be repositioned, and the scout view should be repeated until the lesion is appropriately positioned. When the breast position is deemed satisfactory, the patient's skin should be marked with a felt-tip marker so that any patient movement during the procedure can be readily assessed.

At this point, stereoradiographs are obtained. As explained in Chapters 5 and 9, these images are angled appropriately from the perpendicular in each direction from the central plane. They allow a computer to calculate the lesion's depth from the skin surface. It is important to be certain that the same spot, in the center of the mass, or the same calcification is targeted on both of these views.

For sonographic guidance, or if imaging guidance is not needed because the lesion is palpable, the patient is positioned so that she is comfortable enough to lie still while achieving minimal distance from the skin to the lesion. The breast should be positioned so that it is as immobile as possible. If the lesion is in the outer half of the patient's breast, the patient usually lies in a semidecubitus position, with a pillow in place to support her lower back. The patient usually lies on the side opposite the involved breast. If the lesion is in the medial half of the patient's breasts, the patient usually lies in a supine position.

The patient's skin is wiped with a cotton swab soaked in isopropyl alcohol or Betadine solution. If sonographic or palpation guidance is used, the patient is draped with sterile towels. Enough towels should be used to create an adequate sterile work space to perform the procedure. If desired, the ultrasound transducer also can be draped at this point. This step is not necessary if the transducer has already been disinfected with Betadine, cydex, or alcohol. If a transducer drape is used, enough gel must be placed on both the inside and outside of the transducer cover to allow for optimal contact without interference by air. Sterile gel should be used against the patient's skin.

If desired by the radiologist or the patient, a small amount of local anesthetic may be used. The use of an anesthetic should be limited to the skin surface because the cytologic sample may be diluted by the presence of anesthetic in the sampled area. The anesthetic also may cause damage to the cells themselves.

Needle Placement with Stereotaxic Guidance

The 22-, 23-, or 25-gauge needle should be placed through the skin into the center of the lesion, using the coordinates calculated by the computer. Alternatively, a lower-gauge, outer-guide needle may be placed into the center of the lesion, and the sampling needle may be placed through this guide needle.

To confirm appropriate needle position, stereoradiographs should be obtained at this point (Fig. 7-1). The sampling or guide needle is appropriately positioned if its tip overlies the point that has been targeted within the lesion in both stereoradiographs. If necessary, the needle should be repositioned, and stereoradiographs should be repeated until the needle is appropriately positioned within the lesion on both views.

Needle Placement with Sonographic Guidance

The linear (preferably 7.5 MHz or higher frequency) transducer should be placed on the patient's skin so that both the lesion and the path of the needle are visible (Fig. 7-2A).

The needle should be introduced through the patient's skin and the needle tip directed into the lesion under sonographic visualization (Fig. 7-2B). Alternatively, a low-gauge, outer-guide needle may be placed into the center of the lesion, and the sampling needle may be placed through this guide needle. Adjustment of the needle direction should be made until the echo representing the needle tip clearly lies at or a few millimeters superficial to the edge of the lesion on two orthogonal views.

The needle position should be documented, with sonograms obtained in two orthogonal planes (Fig. 7-2C).

Needle Placement When the Lesion Is Palpable

To place a needle into a palpable breast lesion, the operator should place the fingers of the nondominant hand around the lesion to immobilize it. The needle is introduced through the patient's skin into the lesion. One can usually determine that the needle tip lies within the palpable solid lesion when there is a difference in the amount of resistance to the needle's forward progress. This can be confirmed by releasing the needle and moving the palpable abnormality a few millimeters back and forth. If the needle moves with the lesion, the needle is securely located within the lesion.

Aspiration Technique

Two aspiration techniques have been used successfully in the breast: suction and capillary aspiration. For suction aspiration, a syringe in the resting posi-

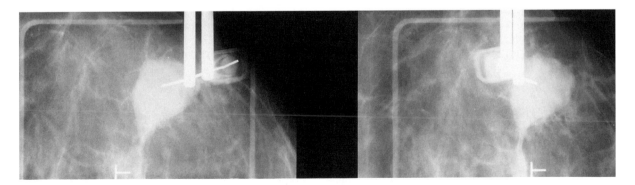

Fig. 7-1. Stereoradiographs after needle placement reveal that the biopsy needle is appropriately situated. Placement can be determined because the tip of the needle overlies the same portion of the lesion on both images. As shown in this example, the first pass through a mass should be through the center of the lesion.

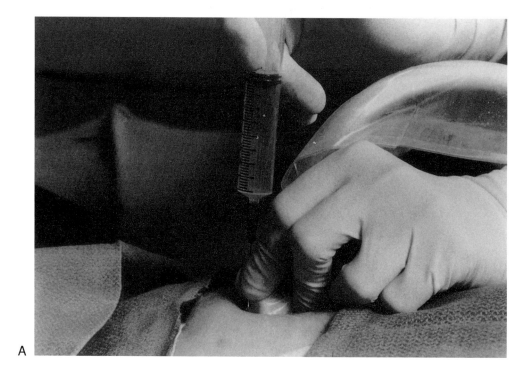

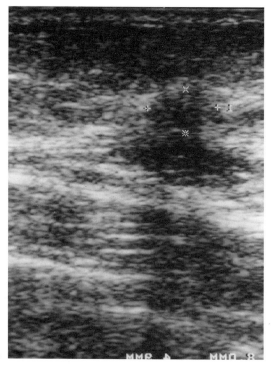

Fig. 7-2. (A) During sonographically guided FNAB, the draped transducer is held in one hand while the needle is introduced into the nonpalpable lesion with the other. **(B)** In this case the needle is introduced so it extends along the long axis of the linear transducer after the transducer is positioned directly over the lesion. *(Figure continues.)*

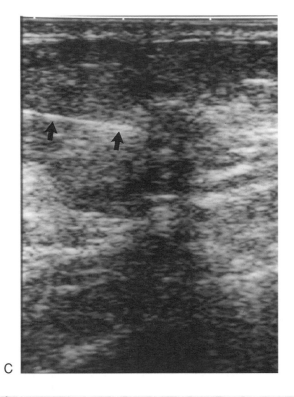

C

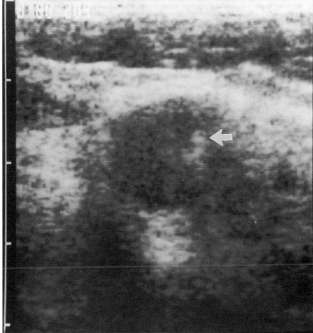

D

Fig. 7-2. *(Continued).* **(C)** In this way, as the needle *(arrows)* approaches the mass from the leading edge of the transducer, it can be followed a considerable distance before it enters the lesion, and its direction can be adjusted, if necessary. **(D)** After penetrating the mass, an orthogonal image can be obtained to confirm that the needle *(arrow)* actually traverses the lesion.

tion is attached to the sampling needle. If desired, a syringe holder and/or tubing may be attached to the syringe. Suction is applied by pulling the plunger of the syringe 5 to 20 cc, depending on the size of the syringe. This maneuver can be accomplished through the use of tubing if an assistant is available, or through the use of a syringe holder or pistol.

For capillary aspiration, attached syringe or tubing is not used and suction is not applied. Some authors have reported that this technique provides a similar cellular yield to suction aspiration without the amount of bleeding into the specimen that can make FNAB interpretation somewhat more difficult. [13,14]

For both aspiration techniques, the sampling needle should be moved back and forth rapidly within the lesion. The needle should be angled in multiple directions so as to sample a small cone within the lesion (Fig. 7-3).

For the suction aspiration technique, suction should be maintained until some material appears in the transparent plastic needle hub, or for at least 20 up-and-down motions in varying directions if no material is seen in the hub. (Getting visible material

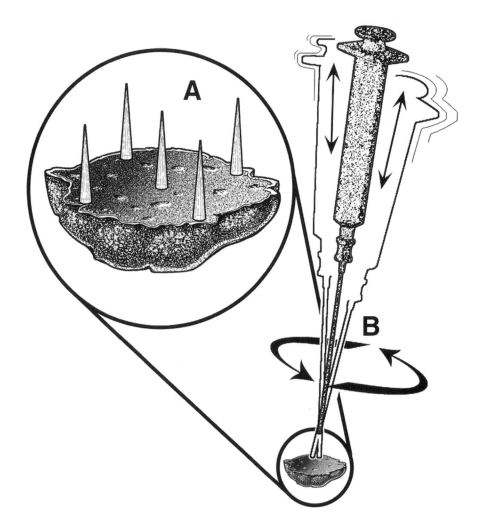

Fig. 7-3. When sampling a lesion with FNAB, as much of the lesion as possible should be needled. **(A)** Multiple sites within a solid mass should be targeted, including the center and uniformly spaced areas in the periphery. **(B)** As the needle passes through these areas both translational and rotational motions are used as continuous suction is applied on the syringe plunger. Rotation of the needle improves the dislodgment of cellular material. Redirecting the needle in a fan-shaped pattern as it serially passes through each site improves tissue sampling.

into the hub may require as many as 20 or more up-and-down motions of the needle with continuous suction, but this does not guarantee visible material will appear in the hub.) With material in the hub of the needle or after 20 up-and-down movements of the needle, the syringe plunger is released and the sampling needle withdrawn.

For the capillary aspiration technique, the lesion should be sampled with at least 20 up-and-down motions of the needle or for approximately 30 to 45 seconds. This step allows material to accumulate within the lumen of the needle.

After the needle is withdrawn, firm compression should be applied to the patient's breast to reduce the likelihood of hematoma formation.

If a cytopathologist is present for the procedure, he or she can perform the aspiration after the needle is positioned by the radiologist. Ideally, the most experienced person should obtain and smear the specimens, as this technique is operator-dependent. It is useful to practice aspiration and smearing technique with an apple or another piece of fruit before trying it on patients.

Immediate Processing of the Specimen

Ideally, the specimen should be prepared by a trained cytotechnologist or by a cytopathologist. If that is not possible, the radiologist or an assistant should be trained in specimen preparation. Optimally, slides should be made immediately from the aspirated material, with some slides allowed to air dry and some immediately fixed. Alternatively, but less optimally, all material can be placed in a rinse solution for later spinning and smearing in the cytology laboratory.

Fully frosted or "plus" slides are intended to be used with fixative. Clear, nonfrosted glass slides are intended to be air dried. The slides should be labeled and laid out before the aspiration so that the specimen can be smeared as soon as it is aspirated. Cytologic specimens tend to dry quickly if not smeared. It is possible to damage the specimen, rendering it uninterpretable, if the specimen dries before smearing. Generally, at least four slides are needed per needle pass. More can be made if desired. Usually one fixed slide is all that is needed per pass, and it is generally the first slide prepared.

If slides are to be prepared in the radiology department, an air-filled syringe should be attached to the sampling needle, and the needle should be placed bevel-side down against the slides (Fig. 7-4). Care should be taken to place only one drop of material on each slide. If the same needle is to be reused on subsequent passes, the needle should be placed as close as possible to the slide so as to minimize loss of the aspirated material.

Two smearing techniques are acceptable: the blood smear technique and the compression technique. The blood smear technique is also used for preparing peripheral blood smears. The first fully frosted or plus slide is smeared using a second nonfrosted clear glass slide. This is accomplished by inverting the second (clear) slide on top of the drop that had been placed on the first fully frosted or plus slide. For the compression smear technique, the second slide is dropped squarely onto the first slide so that the material on the first slide spreads out across the slides evenly. For both techniques, when the drop spreads across the slides, the slides are gently slid (not pulled) apart (Fig. 7-5). The slide used for smearing the drops can be air dried and used for interpretation, resulting in four to six slides per pass submitted for review.

The fully frosted or plus slides should be fixed immediately by immersing them in 95 percent alcohol, in 50 percent alcohol/50 percent water solution, or by using a spray fixative (Fig. 7-6). The nonfrosted, clear glass slides should be allowed to air dry. (Fig. 7-7).

After all slides from a pass are made, the material remaining in the needle should be placed into a rinse solution for later spinning and smearing (Fig. 7-8). Acceptable rinse solutions include a solution of 50 percent Ringer's lactate/50 percent alcohol, Cytolyt, or any balanced salt solution. If a balanced salt solution is used for the rinse, it should be sent to the cytology laboratory as soon as possible for immediate processing so that excessive cellular damage does not occur. The needle may be rinsed once after all passes are made if the same sampling needle is used for all passes.

Repeat Sampling

If a cytopathologist within the breast imaging suite is immediately available to interpret the specimen, it is possible that only one pass is necessary to obtain diagnostic material. In general, the cytopathologist

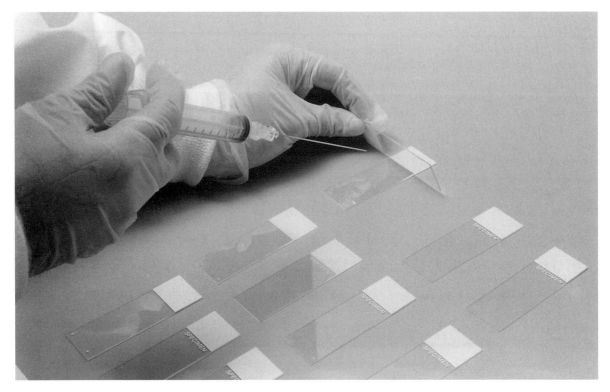

Fig. 7-4. When depositing material on the cytology slide, a second slide can be used to prevent splattering. Ideally, only a single drop of material should be placed on each slide.

determines the need for further samples from the same lesion. This might require five or more passes into the lesion. These passes should be made into different parts of the lesion, to different calcifications within a cluster, or as directed by the on-site cytopathologist.

If a cytopathologist is not available for immediate interpretation, it is good practice to make at least four or five passes into each lesion being sampled. These passes should be made into different parts of the lesion. Ideally, the first pass should be made into the center of the lesion. Subsequent passes should be made at 12, 3, 6, and 9 o'clock positions for spherical lesions. For oblong lesions, the second through fifth specimens should be obtained within the lesion along the radii extending to 12, 3, 6, and 9 o'clock.

If the coaxial method of lesion sampling is used, the outer guide needle should be repositioned so that the sampling needle can be moved into the most superficial aspect of the lesion for pass 2 and the deepest aspect of the lesion for pass 3. Passes 4 and 5 should be made after repositioning the guide nee-

dle into another part of the lesion and positioning the sampling needle in the superficial and deep aspects of the lesion within the new plane. More than five passes can be made if visual inspection of the specimen suggests that it is inadequate.

Processing the Specimen in the Cytology Laboratory

All slides and rinse solutions should be sent to the cytology laboratory as soon as possible after the procedure to allow for optimal preservation of diagnostic material. The cytopathologist should place all bloody smears in Carnoy's solution or water for approximately 5 minutes before staining to lyse the red blood cells present in the specimen. Air-dried slides should be stained using either Diff-Quik or Romanowsky methods. Fixed slides should be stained with Papanicolaou or hematoxylin and eosin methods. Millipore filters or cytospin smears should be prepared from the rinse solution and stained with the Papanicolaou method.

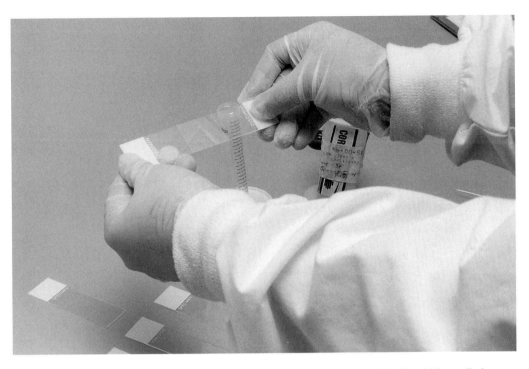

Fig. 7-5. After a drop of specimen has been deposited on a slide, a second slide should be pulled very gently over the first to prepare the smear. It is important to gently slide, not pull, the slides apart.

FNAB INTERPRETATION

In general, cytopathologists use a 4-point scale to interpret cytologic material. Diagnostic categories include benign, atypical, probably malignant, and malignant (Figs. 7-9 and 7-10). Lesions often can be subclassified by type. These subclassifications include lobular neoplasia, lobular hyperplasia, lobular carcinoma, ductal hyperplasia, ductal carcinoma (e.g., cribriform and micropapillary subtypes), sclerosing adenosis, fat necrosis, apocrine metaplasia, fibroadenoma, intraductal papilloma, and duct ectasia. In addition, a specimen can be considered insufficient for diagnosis, usually if it contains only fat or fibrous tissue, or if fewer than six epithelial fragments are present.

ACCURACY AND INADEQUATE SAMPLE RATE

For FNAB, agreement between the pathologist's interpretation of the histologic information obtained through open surgical biopsy and the cytologic material obtained percutaneously has varied from 80 to 92

percent.[15,16] Stereotaxically and sonographically guided FNAB also is limited by the frequent occurrence of insufficient specimens. These have occurred in 0 to 28 percent of FNAB samples of nonpalpable lesions.[15–21] Even when FNAB is performed on surgical specimens, the inadequate sample rate is 7 percent.[22]

When adequate cytologic sampling is obtained, however, very few false-positive results occur when compared to open biopsy, with specificities and positive predictive values both reported between 91 and 100 percent. More important, when adequate cytologic material is obtained, sensitivities have been reported between 83 and 100 percent, and negative predictive values have ranged between 50 and 100 percent.[15–17,19,20,23–26] These percentages vary among centers, depending on the level of cytologic interpretation considered positive; for example, atypia was considered negative by some and positive by others.[15,20] The percentages also have varied depending on the type of mammographic lesion being sampled. Data regarding which types of lesions are best sampled with this technique, however, are limited because the numbers of reported cases of each type that have been evaluated at each center are too small.[19]

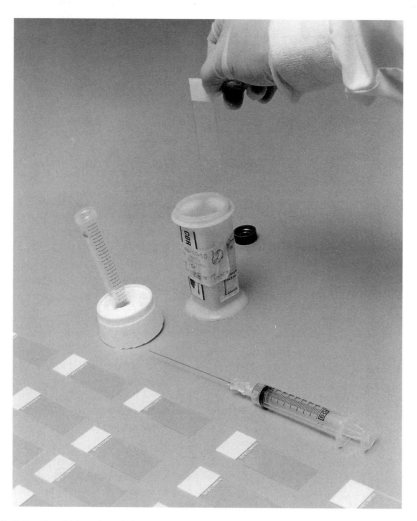

Fig. 7-6. Fixed slides should be placed directly into fixative solution, as described in the text. The container of fixative with slides can then be transported to the cytology laboratory.

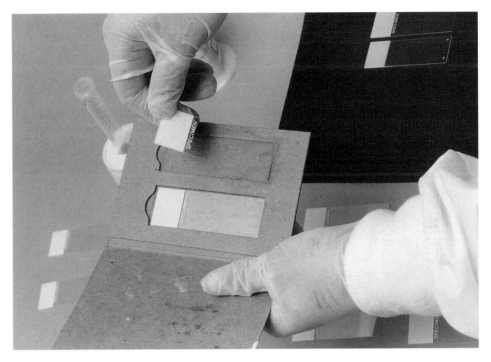

Fig. 7-7. The air-dried slides can be placed in reusable slide boxes for transport to the cytology laboratory. Note that all slides should be labeled with appropriate patient information.

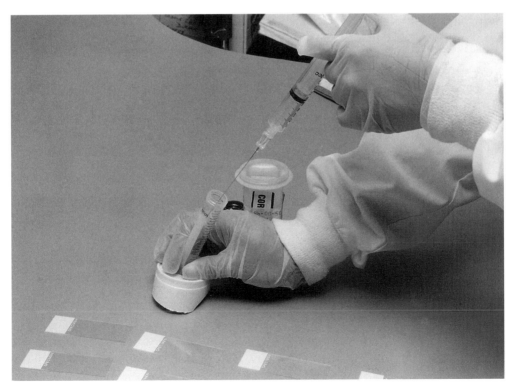

Fig. 7-8. After all of the slides are prepared, the remaining material is placed into a rinse solution, as described in the text. A small amount of the rinse solution should be aspirated up into the needle and syringe and then replaced into the solution. The same tube of rinse solution can be used for all passes into the same lesion. If more than one lesion is sampled, specimens should be submitted separately and should include information identifying each biopsy site.

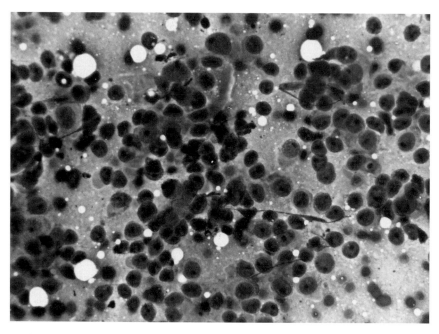

Fig. 7-9. A typical cytologic specimen interpreted as malignant. This air-dried Diff-Quik-stained slide ($\times$ 200), reveals ductal carcinoma. Features that suggest malignancy are the high cellularity and the discohesiveness of the cells. In addition, the cells themselves have a high nuclear/cytoplasmic ratio and large nuclei with prominent nucleoli. (Photomicrograph courtesy of Susan Maygarden, M.D., Department of Pathology, University of North Carolina–Chapel Hill.)

MANAGEMENT DECISIONS BASED ON FNAB AND MAMMOGRAPHY RESULTS

It is important to correlate FNAB results with mammographic findings when deciding whether follow-up mammography or histologic confirmation is indicated.[27] This correlation is relatively straightforward when the suspicion of malignancy from the mammographic findings is high and the FNAB is interpreted as probably malignant or malignant. Clearly, a surgical procedure (excisional biopsy or lumpectomy) is indicated in these cases. Likewise, if the probability of malignancy from the mammographic appearance is low (lesions that are probably benign or indeterminate) and the FNAB results are definitively benign and suggestive of a benign diagnosis such as a fibroadenoma, follow-up mammography, either at 6 months or 1 year, would be preferable to open surgical biopsy. Diagnoses that can be made with this technology that can be followed up with mammography when the mammographic findings are supportive of them include fibroadenoma, lymph node, fat necrosis, papilloma, and nonproliferative fibrocystic change without atypia.

It is also clear that a benign FNAB interpretation in the setting of probably malignant or malignant mammographic findings should be followed by histologic evaluation of the lesion. As with suspicious palpable lesions, a benign FNAB is not that reassuring in this setting, as there is always the possibility of a sampling error. Similarly, if the mammographic probability of malignancy is relatively low and the FNAB results are probably malignant or malignant, histologic confirmation may be indicated before definitive surgical therapy to avoid the consequence of excessive surgical intervention. An FNAB interpretation of atypical cytology also justifies further histologic evaluation for any type of palpable or nonpalpable lesion.

In addition, an inadequate FNAB specimen should be treated as if no information has been obtained. That is, if the lesion was suspicious enough by physical examination or mammography to warrant needle aspiration, insufficient sampling of the lesion by FNAB should be followed by repeat cytologic or histologic sampling. Failure to obtain an adequate specimen on the first attempt at tissue sampling does not diminish the need for analysis of cells from the lesion in question.

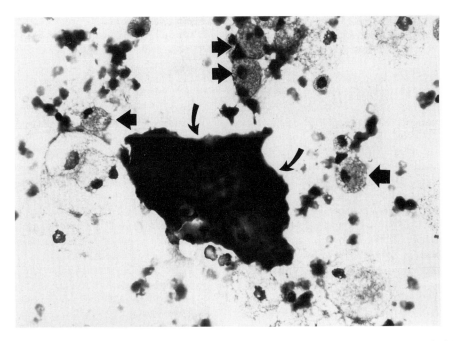

Fig. 7-10. A typical cytologic specimen interpreted as benign. This air-dried Diff-Quik-stained slide (× 200) suggests fibrocystic change. Features that suggest this diagnosis are the presence of benign foam cells (*straight arrows*) and the cohesive sheet of benign-appearing ductal epithelium (*curved arrows*). The cells themselves appear benign because the nuclei are small and regular. (Photomicrograph courtesy of Susan Maygarden, M.D., Department of Pathology, University of North Carolina–Chapel Hill.)

COMPLICATIONS AND RISKS

The most frequent acute complications of breast FNAB are fainting and hematoma formation; fortunately, neither are common.[18,19,28] The only other potential complication that has been reported is seeding of the needle track by malignant cells. The risk of this complication in FNAB is about 0.005 percent.[29]

FNAB can produce mammographic changes that may be confused with malignancy. The rate of postaspiration hematoma formation visible on mammography has varied from 6 to 30 percent.[30] This problem can be rectified readily by performing mammographic imaging before placing any needles in the breast. This recommendation is important for referring clinicians who desire evaluation of palpable abnormalities. The breast imaging clinic must accommodate immediate imaging of women with palpable lesions so that the diagnostic test (e.g., FNAB) can be performed in a timely fashion.

SUMMARY

When skilled cytopathologists are available, FNAB can contribute significantly to the management of palpable and nonpalpable breast lesions. This procedure is quite dependent on both the interpretative and aspiration skills of the operators. Before providing this service to patients, radiologists should work closely with their local cytopathologist so that the results are likely to correlate well with the histopathologic truth. When used judiciously and carefully in appropriate circumstances, FNAB can save money and reduce patient morbidity.

REFERENCES

1. Feig SA. Decreased breast cancer mortality through mammographic screening: results of clinical trials. Radiology 1988; 167:659–665.
2. Schwartz G, Feig S, Patchefsky A. Significance and staging of nonpalpable carcinomas of the breast. Surg Gynecol Obstet 1988; 166:6–10.
3. Sickles EA. Periodic mammographic follow-up of probably benign lesions: results in 3,184 consecutive cases. Radiology 1991; 179:463–468.
4. Sickles EA. Nonpalpable, circumscribed, noncalcified solid breast masses: likelihood of malignancy based on lesion size and age of patient. Radiology 1994; 192: 439–442.

5. Helvie MA, Ikeda DM, Adler DD. Localization and needle aspiration of breast lesions: complications in 370 cases. Am J Roentgenol 1991; 157:711–714.
6. Cyrlak D. Induced costs of low-cost screening mammography. Radiology 1988; 168:661–663.
7. Eddy DM, Hasselblad V, McGwney W, Hendee WR. The value of mammography screening in women under age 50 years. JAMA 1988; 259:1512–1519.
8. Ciatto S, Catarzi S, Morrone D, et al. Fine-needle aspiration cytology of nonpalpable breast lesions: US versus stereotaxic guidance. Radiology 1993; 188:195–198.
9. Mitnick JS, Vazquez MF, Roses DF, et al. Stereotaxic localization for fine-needle aspiration breast biopsy. Initial experience with 300 patients. Arch Surg 1991; 126:1137–1140.
10. O'Malley F, Casey T, Winfield A, et al. Clinical correlates of false-negative fine needle aspirations of the breast in a consecutive series of 1,005 patients. Surg Gynecol Obstet 1993; 176:360–364.
11. Lofgren M, Andersson I, Lindholm K. Stereotactic, x-ray guided, fine needle aspiration biopsy of nonpalpable breast lesions: comparison with the coordinating grid localization technique. Recent Results Cancer Res 1990; 119:100-104.
12. Svane G, Silfversward C. Stereotaxic needle biopsy of non-palpable breast lesions. Cytologic and histopathologic findings. Acta Radiol Diagn (Stockh) 1983; 4:283–288.
13. Zajdela A, Zillhardt P, Voillemot N. Cytological diagnosis by fine needle sampling without aspiration. Cancer 1987; 59:1201–1205.
14. Fornage BD, Sneige N, Singletary SE. Masses in breasts with implants: diagnosis with US-guided fine-needle aspiration biopsy. Radiology 1994; 191:339–342.
15. Fajardo L, Davis J, Wiens J, Trego D. Mammography guided stereotactic fine-needle aspiration cytology of nonpalpable breast lesions. Am J Roentgenol 1990; 155:977–981.
16. Dowlatshahi K, Gent H, Schmidt R, et al. Nonpalpable breast tumor: diagnosis with stereotactic localization and fine-needle aspiration. Radiology 1989; 170:427–433.
17. Dowlatshahi K, Yaremko L, Kluskens L, Jokich P. Nonpalpable breast lesions: findings of stereotactic needle core biopsy and fine-needle aspiration cytology. Radiology 1991; 181:745–750.
18. Azavedo E, Svane G, Auer G. Stereotactic fine-needle biopsy in 2594 mammographically detected nonpalpable lesions. Lancet 1989; 1033–1035.
19. Lofgren M, Anderson I, Lindholm K. Stereotactic fine-needle aspiration for cytologic diagnosis of nonpalpable breast lesions. Am J Roentgenol 1990; 154:1191–1195.
20. Ciatto S, Rosselli del Turco M, Bravetti P. Nonpalpable breast lesions: stereotactic fine-needle aspiration cytology. Radiology 1989; 173:57–59.
21. Arishita G, Cruz BK, Harding C, Arbutina D. Mammogram-directed fine-needle aspiration of nonpalpable breast lesions. J Surg Oncol 1991; 48:153–157.
22. Teixidor H, Wojtasek D, Reiches E, et al. Fine-needle aspiration breast biopsy specimens: correlation of histologic and cytologic findings. Radiology 1992; 184:55–58.
23. Bibbo M, Scheiber M, Cajulis R, et al. Stereotactic fine-needle aspiration. Cytology of clinically occult malignant and premalignant breast lesions. Acta Cytol 1988; 32:193–201.
24. Fornage BD, Faroux MJ, Simatos A. Breast masses: US-guided fine-needle aspiration biopsy. Radiology 1987; 162:409–411.
25. Gordon PB, Goldenberg SL, Chan NHL. Solid breast lesions: diagnosis with US-guided fine-needle aspiration biopsy. Radiology 1993; 189:573–580.
26. Benedetto J, Allora V, Wyatt L. Accuracy of fine-needle aspiration biopsy in diagnosis of palpable breast masses: two-year results of a university-affiliated community hospital. J Am Osteopath Assoc 1993; 93:585–587.
27. Jackson V, Reynolds H. Stereotaxic needle-core biopsy and fine-needle aspiration cytologic evaluation of nonpalpable breast lesions. Radiology 1991; 181:633–634.
28. Evans WP, Cade SH. Needle localization and fine-needle aspiration biopsy of nonpalpable breast lesions with use of standard and stereotactic equipment. Radiology 1989; 173:53–56.
29. Smith EH. The hazards of fine-needle aspiration biopsy. US Med Biol 1984; 10:629–634.
30. Horobin JM, Matthew BM, Preece PE, Thompson AJ. Effects of fine needle aspiration on subsequent mammograms. Br J Surg 1992; 79:52–54.

8 PERCUTANEOUS BIOPSY OF NONPALPABLE BREAST LESIONS: CORE OR FINE NEEDLE ASPIRATION

D. David Dershaw

Percutaneous needle biopsy of the breast can be performed using two different biopsy techniques: fine needle aspiration biopsy (FNAB) or large-bore core biopsy. The radiologist must decide which technique to use before performing percutaneous breast biopsies. The manner by which each of these procedures is performed has been discussed in detail in the preceding two chapters. This chapter discusses the advantages and disadvantages of each technique. The decision about which to use depends on the equipment available, the experience of the physician performing the biopsy, and the availability of pathology expertise in interpreting different types of specimens. It may be useful to be able to perform both types of biopsies and to use different techniques in various situations. At Memorial Sloan-Kettering Cancer Center, New York, we usually opt for large-bore (14-gauge) core biopsy, but occasionally, we find it useful to perform FNAB.

FINE NEEDLE ASPIRATION BIOPSY

FNAB can be performed using sonographic, mammographic, or stereotaxic imaging to guide the needle into the breast. A small-gauge needle (20-gauge or higher) is used to obtain the specimen. The needle and syringe used in the biopsy are available in any radiology department. Local anesthetic may be given, but is not necessary. Multiple passes must be made to obtain the specimen, which is smeared on glass slides or deposited in a container filled with an appropriate fixative. When the specimen is placed on slides, cytologic interpretation can be made immediately to determine whether the specimen is adequate and whether the area sampled is benign or malignant. To obtain this information immediately, however, a cytologist or cytopathologist must be in the room at the time the FNAB is performed. Otherwise, the adequacy of the specimen and the diagnosis are determined later. Complications are few, but a significant hematoma can result.

Data from various studies using FNAB have revealed its advantages and disadvantages. Sensitivity for this technique has ranged from 0.68 to 0.93; its specificity has ranged from 0.88 to 1.00.[1] These numbers usually represent only those patients for whom the procedure resulted in an adequate specimen. When a sufficient sampling has resulted from FNAB, cytologic analysis is usually reliable. The best results for FNAB, however, have been reported when an experienced cytopathologist is present at the time of the biopsy. In one series of 9,533 breast FNABs performed in Italy, the inadequacy rate in the entire group was 20.8 percent.[2] The incidence was greatest (32.4 percent) among those who had performed the fewest numbers of FNABs (less than 200). Those who had performed the procedure most often (more than 400 times) still had an insufficient sampling rate of 19.7 percent. In addition, although the sensitivity rate in this series was 90.1 percent for invasive cancer, it fell to 79.6 percent for in situ cancers. When using FNAB, it is desirable to have a cytopathologist present during the procedure to assess whether the sample is sufficient, as multiple samplings may be necessary to obtain a specimen that is adequate for diagnosis.

The ability to perform FNAB of the breast well is experience dependent. As is evident from the preceding data, the procedure may need to be performed several hundred times before a radiologist becomes proficient at it. This technique is not highly automated, but rather depends on the physician's ability to direct the needle into the lesion in question and dislodge cells from the area.

The accuracy of FNAB is comparable regardless of the imaging technique used, as long as an adequate specimen is obtained. In a comparison of FNAB performed with sonographic and stereotaxic guidance, there was no significant difference in the biopsy results.[3] Insufficient sampling rates were a problem with some lesions. For example, 32 percent of smoothly marginated masses could not be adequately sampled. Although results were comparable with both types of imaging, the procedure was completed more quickly and inexpensively using sonographic guidance. Another study using FNAB with radiographic guidance found that when an adequate specimen was obtained, the diagnosis of malignancy could be made with a specificity of 94 percent and a sensitivity of 97 percent; however, the aspirates were inadequate in 54 percent of the cases.[4]

Complications are rare. Hematomas may result, but they usually resolve spontaneously. The only medically significant complication is pneumothorax, which can occur in 1 in 1,000 to 1 in 10,000 procedures.[5]

Histologic assessment of the FNAB specimen is somewhat limited. Cytologic reporting includes a "suspicious" category in which an absolute diagnosis of benign or malignant is not made. When a specimen is read as malignant, cytologic evaluation cannot determine whether the cancer is invasive. Most lesions that are biopsied are benign, but the cytologic analysis may only read "benign," making it difficult to be certain whether cells obtained were from the lesion in question or from adjacent normal breast tissue. Analysis of the FNAB specimen requires a cytopathologist who is trained in breast cytology. In institutions where this expertise is not available, FNAB cannot be performed or the specimen needs to be sent elsewhere for interpretation.

FNAB is ideally performed by a physician experienced at this procedure with a breast cytopathologist present in the room, so that the specimen can be evaluated for adequacy as well as diagnosis. This protocol ensures that the patient will not require repeat biopsy and enables the radiologist to give the patient a diagnosis immediately. Sonographic, stereotaxic, or radiographic imaging can be used. Complications are rare, and the procedure is inexpensive to perform.

LARGE-BORE CORE BIOPSY

Large-bore core biopsy of the breast is a newer procedure than FNAB, and therefore the accuracy of the technique is not as well documented. The procedure is performed with a cutting needle measuring at least 18 gauge; a 14-gauge needle is always used at many institutions. In addition to a special cutting needle, equipment required includes a biopsy gun. A local anesthetic is given as part of the procedure. Imaging can be done with stereotaxic or sonographic equipment. Complications are rare.

Variations in technique are important in determining the success of the procedure in making a diagnosis. Smaller core and shorter throw needles are not as accurate as larger gauge, longer throw needles.[6] Accuracies have been reported at more than 90 percent by several investigators.[7-9] False-positive results have not been a problem, but false-negative results are reported, as they are with FNAB.

Insufficient sampling is rarely a problem in women undergoing core biopsy for mass lesions. In some instances, however, a well-defined mass in fatty tissue, particularly a fibroadenoma, may be deflected by the cutting needle. Successful biopsy may be more difficult in this situation than with other solid lesions. Under stereotaxic guidance, calcifications may be more difficult to biopsy successfully than masses.[10] To assess adequacy of sampling, specimen radiography should be used.

Histologic analysis of the core of tissue obtained with core biopsy technique requires tissue processing, as with a surgical specimen, and results are not available for a day or more after the biopsy. No immediate answer can be given to the patient. Definitive diagnoses are usually possible in benign disease, allowing the radiologist to be certain that the appropriate site in the breast was biopsied.

When a cancerous lesion is biopsied, more detailed information can be obtained with core biopsy than with FNAB. Whereas FNAB can determine only whether a lesion is malignant, core biopsy can often determine whether the cancer is invasive and, therefore, requires an axillary lymph node dissection as part of the surgical treatment. It is not possible to reliably make a diagnosis of in situ cancer based on core biopsy because sampling error may have missed the invasive component of the tumor. Hormone receptor analysis is also possible with core biopsy specimens.

Because core biopsy removes a significant volume of tissue, it is possible that small lesions can be totally excised with core biopsy. If the lesion is benign, this is not of clinical importance. With malignant lesions, however, surgical re-excision of the area is necessary. If the cancer has been totally removed, it may no longer be possible to identify the area of the breast requiring re-excision. Small lesions (5 mm or less in diameter), therefore, may be inappropriate for core biopsy.

Although core biopsy is a longer procedure than FNAB and may not be as well tolerated by some patients, it probably has a complication rate comparable to FNAB. In addition to bleeding, which is rarely clinically significant, and pneumothorax, milk fistula formation has been reported in a lactating woman.[11] We have been hesitant to perform core biopsy in women with breast augmentation prostheses for fear of rupturing the implant. This complication may also occur with FNAB. As a local anesthetic needs to be instilled in the area of the breast undergoing core biopsy, an allergic reaction to the anesthetic is always a possibility; therefore, allergy to local anesthetic is a contraindication for core biopsy.

Whereas data have indicated a significant learning curve for performing FNAB, core biopsy of the breast, particularly when performed with stereotaxic guidance, is highly automated and more easily performed successfully with far less experience. Sonographically guided biopsy, however, is probably more operator dependent and requires significant sonographic skill and dexterity. Sonographically guided core biopsy also is often performed using two sets of hands, the radiologist's to position the needle and the technologist's to fire the gun.

CHOOSING THE APPROPRIATE TECHNIQUE

Which biopsy technique should be used in patient care? The answer depends on the equipment available and the skills of the radiologists in the practice. At Memorial Sloan-Kettering Cancer Center, we routinely use core biopsy, whenever possible. The biopsy is performed either with sonographic guidance or a dedicated, prone stereotaxic table. We believe that more histologic information is obtained from the biopsy with the larger tissue sample obtained in a core sampling. When a women is diagnosed with invasive cancer on core biopsy, the patient and her surgeon can plan a definitive surgical procedure with axillary nodal dissection; no additional surgical biopsy is necessary. In women who are being biopsied for calcifications, specimen radiography allows confirmation that an adequate sample has been obtained, as would occur during surgical biopsy.

As at other centers, insufficient sampling has been a significant problem with FNAB at our Center, where a cytopathologist is not present in the room when FNABs are performed. Although this problem is obviated by performing core sampling, we are unable to provide patients with results on the same day as the procedure.

We do not perform core biopsy on women who cannot tolerate a long procedure. Core biopsy takes about 20 minutes to 1 hour to perform; FNAB can be accomplished in a few minutes. In addition, patients who are allergic to local anesthetic cannot undergo core biopsy. Women who have been augmented are preferentially biopsied with FNAB because of the fear of perforating the prosthesis.

Occasionally, we will opt to perform FNAB rather than core biopsy. This choice is usually made when a cyst aspiration is being performed to evaluate what has appeared to be a "dirty" cyst sonographically. These lesions will sometimes be found to be solid.

Because a fine needle has been introduced for the cyst aspiration, these procedures are readily converted into FNAB tissue samplings.

REFERENCES

1. Fajardo LL, Jackson VP, Hunter TB. Interventional procedures in diseases of the breast: needle biopsy, pneumocystography, and galactography. Am J Roentgenol 1992; 158:1231–1238.
2. Ciatto S, Cariaggi P, Bulgaresi P et al. Fine needle aspiration cytology of the breast: review of 9533 consecutive cases. Breast 1993; 2:87–90.
3. Ciatto S, Cataarzi S, Morrone D, Del Turco MR. Fine-needle aspiration cytology of nonpalpable breast lesions: US versus stereotaxic guidance. Radiology 1993; 188: 195–198.
4. Helvie MA, Baker DE, Adler DD et al. Radiographically guided fine-needle aspiration of nonpalpable breast lesions. Radiology 1990; 174:657–661.
5. Catania S, Veronesi P, Marassi A et al. Risk of pneumothorax after fine needle aspiration of the breast: Italian experience of more than 200,000 aspirations. Breast 1993; 2:246–247.
6. Parker SH. When is core biopsy really core? Radiology 1992; 185:641–642.
7. Elvecrog EL, Lechner MC, Nelson MT. Nonpalpable breast lesions: correlation of stereotaxic large-core needle biopsy and surgical biopsy results. Radiology 1993; 188:453–455.
8. Parker SH, Lovin JD, Jobe WE et al. Stereotactic breast biopsy with a biopsy gun. Radiology 1990; 176:741–747.
9. Dronkers DJ. Stereotaxic core biopsy of breast lesions. Radiology 1992; 183:631–634.
10. Liberman L, Evans WP III, Dershaw DD et al. Radiography of microcalcifications in stereotaxic mammary core biopsy vs specimens. Radiology 1994; 190: 223–225.
11. Schackmuth EM, Harlow CL, Norton LW. Milk fistula: a complication after core breast biopsy. Am J Roentgenol 1993; 161:961–962.

9
STEREOTAXIC BIOPSY TECHNIQUE

Laura Liberman

The first description of a stereotaxic breast biopsy device was made in Sweden in the 1970s.[1] Since then, stereotaxic biopsy has been used increasingly in breast diagnosis.[2-14] With appropriate technique, needle biopsy under stereotaxic guidance can provide an accurate, less invasive, and less expensive alternative to surgical biopsy for mammographically evident lesions of the breast that are indeterminate or suspicious for malignancy.

PRINCIPLES OF STEREOTAXIS

The primary principle of stereotaxis is that the location of a lesion in three dimensions can be determined by analyzing the change in position of the lesion on angled views.[1] This three-dimensional information is calculated in terms of the x, y, and z coordinates of the lesion; for patients undergoing biopsy in the prone position, the x axis is horizontal, y is vertical, and z is the depth of the lesion.

The stereotaxic images are obtained by moving the x-ray tube an equal distance to the right and left of midline. Manufacturers have established this to be +15 and −15 degrees along the horizontal or x axis. In some equipment, not only does the angle of the x-ray beam change from the first to the second stereotaxic image, but the location of the image receptor also shifts along the x axis. Two reference points are selected at the level of the back breast support and appear on each stereotaxic image.

The x position of the lesion is equal to the mean of the x positions of the lesion on the two stereotaxic images. Because the change in the direction of the x-ray beam occurs only along the x axis, the y position is constant on the two images and is equal to the true y position of the lesion. The depth of the lesion from the back breast support (Δz) is a function of the displacement of the lesion relative to the displacement of the reference points (Δx) as follows:[15]

$$\Delta z = \frac{\Delta x}{2 \tan (15°)} = 1.866\ \Delta x$$

Because of the mathematical relationships between lesion displacement and lesion location, obtaining the stereotaxic images allows calculation of the precise location of the lesion in three dimensions.

EQUIPMENT

Equipment necessary for performing stereotaxic biopsy is shown in Table 9-1. Instrumentation choices include the use of fine needle aspiration versus core needle biopsy, prone dedicated or upright add-on equipment, and film-screen versus digital mammography. The first issue has been discussed in the preceding four chapters. Relevant aspects of the latter two issues are reviewed here.

107

Table 9-1. STEREOTAXIC BIOPSY EQUIPMENT

For All Procedures

Stereotaxic unit
Sterile gloves
Sterile gauze
Sterile needle holders
Alcohol and/or hydrogen peroxide
Betadine
Lidocaine (1%)
Syringes (5 cc)
Needles (25-gauge, 3/4 in)
Microscope slides

For Core Biopsy

Scalpel (No. 11 straight edge)
Automated gun
Biopsy needle (14-gauge)
Formalin (10% neutral buffered)
Steri-strips (1/4 in)

For Fine Needle Aspiration

Syringes (10 cc)
Needles (22-gauge spinal)
Connecting tubing
95% alcohol

Upright Versus Prone Dedicated Equipment

Two options are currently utilized for stereotaxic biopsy. These are discussed and illustrated in Chapter 5. Briefly, upright units can be added to already existing mammography equipment. Unlike a prone table, which occupies an entire room, the upright units are easily removed from the conventional mammography unit to which they are attached, allowing the room to be used for routine mammography as well as stereotaxic biopsy. Upright, add-on units also allow better access to the posterior breast near the chest wall, as well as to the axilla.

Use of the upright equipment, however, also has several disadvantages. The patient must maintain a sitting position during the biopsy procedure, which is more apt to result in patient movement than the prone position. Work space may be somewhat limited, particularly for performing core biopsy. The patient is able to see the procedure, which may be difficult psychologically and may increase the likelihood of vasovagal reactions. Caines et al.[16] illustrated some of these difficulties in a series of core biopsies performed on upright equipment. Sampling was "problematic," with discordance between mammo-

graphic and histologic findings, lack of sampling of calcifications, or patient motion in 31 (12 percent) of 254 cases.

With a dedicated stereotaxic table, the patient lies in the prone position during the biopsy procedure. The breast is in the dependent position and is placed through an opening in the table. The prone dedicated units are substantially more expensive than the upright add-on equipment. Furthermore, the size of the equipment limits the use of the room in which it is placed. Another problem with the prone-dedicated units is difficulty gaining access to lesions near the chest wall or in the axilla. However, the prone units have several advantages over upright, add-on systems. The table provides a physical barrier between the patient's head and the working area. This barrier is helpful psychologically for the patient, who cannot watch the actual biopsy procedure take place. This barrier probably minimizes vasovagal reactions, and if such reactions do occur, the patient is already lying down. Patient motion is less likely to occur with the patient lying down than with the patient sitting. The prone tables provide more work space, which is particularly important in core needle biopsy.

Results of several studies correlating stereotaxic core biopsy and surgical biopsy results are shown in Table 9-2. Concordance between stereotaxic and surgical biopsy results has ranged from 67[8] to 96 percent,[7] with rates of insufficient samples ranging from 0[7,11] to 17 percent.[8] Obtaining multiple core biopsy specimens and utilizing a 14-gauge needle with patients in the prone position have yielded the best results.

Film-Screen Versus Digital Mammography

The ability to acquire and display mammographic images digitally has dramatically improved the capabilities of stereotaxic equipment. The technical aspects of digital imaging have been described in Chapter 5. The main advantage of digital imaging is the decreased time to perform a procedure. Just as digital imaging decreases the time requirements for needle localization procedures by approximately 50 percent,[17] digital imaging reduces the time required for stereotaxic biopsy. This time saving is important because accurate needle placement requires minimal patient motion; the faster the procedure, the less likely that the patient will move. In a series by Parker et

Table 9-2. Stereotaxic Core Breast Biopsy: Results and Instrumentation

Author	# Cases with Surgical Correlation	Concordance Stereo/Surgery	Insufficient	# Passes	Needle	Gun	Equipment
Parker[5]	102	87%	1%	3–4	18G(N=65) 16G(N=9) 14G(N=29)	Short(N=2) Long(N=101)	Upright(N=30) Prone(N=73)
Parker[7]	102	96%	0%	3–4	14G	Long	Prone
Dowlatshahi[8]	250	67–69%[a]	17%	2–3	20G	Short(N=120) Long(N=130)	Prone
Dronkers[10]	53	91%	6%	2	18G	Short	Upright
Elvecrog[11]	100	94%	0%	≥5	14G	Long	Prone
Gisvold[12]	56	80%	2%	<5	14G	Long	Prone
Gisvold[12]	104	90%	0%	≥5	14G	Long	Prone

[a]Range depending on whether lesions for which diagnosis was atypical or suspicious at core and benign at surgery are scored as concordant or discordant.

al.[18] of 305 patients who underwent digital stereotaxic core biopsy, the time required for biopsy averaged 17 minutes. The radiation dose of digital systems is reduced by almost 50 percent of that needed for film-screen systems.

The area of breast exposed is kept to a minimum by the small field of view, which is 5 × 5 cm in currently available equipment. Although helpful in minimizing radiation dose, however, the small field of view can cause problems. For example, large areas of asymmetric parenchyma may be difficult to discern. Subtle parenchymal densities and faint calcifications also may be difficult to appreciate with digital imaging, although they could be seen readily with film-screen mammography.[17] Failure to resolve some faint lesions, especially calcifications, can sometimes be compensated for by increasing the kVp when using digital imaging. Unlike film-screen imaging, in which this change in technique decreases contrast, in digital imaging it increases the signal-to-noise ratio and may improve imaging. Of course, when purchasing a stereotaxic system, the acquisition of digital imaging capability can add significant expense to the purchase of the system.

INDICATIONS AND CONTRAINDICATIONS

Lesion Considerations

Stereotaxic biopsy should be utilized to obtain histologic diagnoses on mammographically evident lesions for which surgical biopsy would otherwise be recommended. "Probably benign" lesions should be evaluated with short-term mammographic follow-up rather than biopsy[19–22] unless tissue sampling is warranted due to unique circumstances (for example, if the patient is planning a pregnancy) or patient anxiety.

A few contraindications to stereotaxic core needle biopsy do not apply to stereotaxic fine needle aspiration. At my institution I do not perform core biopsy on lesions measuring less than 5 mm at the longest dimension, because such a lesion could be entirely removed at the time of core biopsy. If carcinoma were found and the patient were to desire breast conservation, absence of a localizable lesion on the mammogram could make it more difficult for the surgeon to perform the necessary excision to assess for residual disease and to achieve clear margins. Core biopsy is not an option for lesions surrounded by breast volume that is inadequate to accommodate the excursion of the core biopsy needle.

Patient Considerations

Patient considerations are discussed more fully in Chapter 4, but a brief review of factors affecting patient selection is appropriate. Patients with bleeding diatheses or on anticoagulant therapy should not undergo stereotaxic biopsy unless the coagulation status is corrected. Patients who have taken aspirin or nonsteroidal, anti-inflammatory agents within the previous week should not undergo the procedure, because these agents impair platelet function and may lead to bleeding. Inability to tolerate local anesthesia, although rare, is a contraindication for stereotaxic biopsy.

Hypersensitivity to local anesthetics of the amide type (e.g., lidocaine) is particularly uncommon; allergy most often occurs with ester-type agents (e.g., procaine) and is generally limited to structurally similar compounds.[23]

Inability to cooperate with the procedure is also a contraindication for stereotaxic biopsy. Movement disorders such as Parkinson's disease and other conditions may make it difficult for the patient to remain relatively motionless, even for the short time required. Recent abdominal surgery or the presence of a pacemaker on the chest may make the prone position in particular difficult to maintain. Severe arthritis, particularly of the neck and shoulders, may make stereotaxic biopsy uncomfortable for the patient, but would not be an absolute contraindication.

PREBIOPSY PREPARATION

The imaging work-up should be complete before performing stereotaxic biopsy. Additional views or ultrasound may indicate that the area in question represents a benign process or that no lesion exists. Substantial time and expense are saved and unnecessary procedures avoided by making this determination before attempting biopsy. It may be helpful to check the thickness of the compressed breast parenchyma at the time of diagnostic work-up to determine whether breast thickness is adequate to accommodate the movement of the needle during stereotaxic core biopsy. If the procedure is performed on the basis of films performed at another facility, these films should be submitted and reviewed before scheduling the procedure to ensure that the lesion is real, warrants biopsy, and is amenable to sampling under stereotaxic guidance.

The value of routine prophylactic antibiotics for the prevention of local or systemic infection in low-risk procedures such as stereotaxic biopsy has not been demonstrated.[24] If prophylaxis is deemed appropriate in select circumstances such as patients with prosthetic heart valves, reasonable regimens (in the absence of contraindications) may include a first-generation cephalosporin (e.g., cephalexin, 500 mg orally, or cefazolin, 1 g intravenously) or a macrolide (e.g., erythromycin 500 mg orally) one half hour before the procedure, with consideration of a second dose 6 hours after the procedure.[24]

Patients are instructed to avoid aspirin and non-steroidal, anti-inflammatory agents for one week before the procedure, although they may take acetaminophen. No other preparation is necessary.

INFORMED CONSENT; COMPLICATIONS

Informed consent should be obtained for all stereotaxic biopsy procedures. It is helpful to obtain consent in the room where the biopsy will take place to facilitate the explanation of the procedure to the patient. Potential risks of the procedure include bleeding and infection. These complications are rare. In a recent review of 6,152 breast lesions sampled with percutaneous large-core biopsy under stereotaxic or ultrasound guidance, with follow-up data available in 3,765 cases, Parker et al.[25] reported clinically significant complications in six cases (0.2 percent). There were three hematomas requiring surgical drainage and three infections. The patient should be told that mild discomfort and bruising are expected minor complications of sterotaxic biopsy and she should also be informed of the possibility that the stereotaxic biopsy will yield inadequate material or findings for which surgical excision will be indicated. If the needle courses parallel to the chest wall, pneumothorax is not a potential complication of stereotaxic biopsy.

Patients sometimes inquire whether the stereotaxic biopsy will result in long-term changes in their mammograms. In a study of 24 patients who underwent 6-month follow-up mammograms after stereotaxic core breast biopsy, the only changes were the result of tissue sampling (defects in lesions from which tissue was extracted or decrease in the number of calcifications).[26] Parenchymal scarring, architectural distortion, fat necrosis, and other sequelae of surgical biopsy were not observed.[26]

STEREOTAXIC CORE BIOPSY PROCEDURE

An outline of the procedure for stereotaxic large core biopsy is given in Table 9-3. Many of the preliminary steps in selecting approach and targeting the lesion are identical for FNAB and core biopsy. Steps unique to the particular procedure are discussed separately.

Table 9-3. Stereotaxic Core Biopsy Procedure

1. Films reviewed, approach selected
2. Informed consent obtained
3. Preliminary grid-localizing film obtained and skin marked
4. Patient positioned in stereotaxic equipment
5. Scout film obtained; lesion centered in field of view
6. Stereotaxic images obtained
7. Target selected (must be the same point on both images); coordinates obtained and transmitted to biopsy unit
8. Adequacy of breast thickness assessed
9. Skin cleansed with iodine soap
10. Sterile needle holder placed, needle placed in gun, gun fired in air to demonstrate sound to patient, needle cocked to "prefire" mode
11. Gun mounted in holder, x and y coordinates set (manually if not done automatically in No. 7), needle brought to skin surface
12. Local anesthesia given and scalpel incision made
13. Needle placed to appropriate depth ("z" or "z minus pull-back" as desired)
14. Prefire stereotaxic images obtained and adjustments made, if necessary; needle "pulled back" if not done in No. 13; stroke margin checked
15. Gun fired and postfire stereotaxic images obtained
16. Needle removed from breast and sample removed from needle. For masses, sample placed directly into formalin; for calcifications, sample placed on numbered microscope slide for specimen radiography
17. Additional cores as per protocol, with specimen radiography performed for calcifications
18. Specimens sent to pathology laboratory in formalin
19. After last specimen obtained, compression held for 5 to 10 minutes (with ice if necessary), wound cleansed, and bandaging applied.
20. Postbiopsy instructions given; patient told when and by whom she will be contacted with results and given phone number of radiologist who performed the biopsy
21. Radiologist reviews pathology results and correlates these with imaging studies
22. Patient and referring physician notified of results and recommendations, and addendum written to biopsy report

Selecting the Approach

The approach should allow for clear visualization of the lesion. It is usually preferable to choose an approach that requires traversing the shortest distance from skin to lesion. This approach usually allows for greater accuracy in needle placement because a small error in the angle of placement will result in a smaller error in needle placement for lesions close to the needle entry site than for distant lesions. The shortest distance approach also provides

more tissue on the far side of the lesion to accommodate the excursion of the needle. However, the lesion must be deep enough relative to the skin surface selected for the prefire position of the needle tip to be deep to the skin.

Preliminary Grid-Localizing Film

After the approach is selected, it is helpful to obtain a preliminary image with the alpha-numeric grid used for needle localizations (Fig. 9-1). This technique is particularly useful if digital equipment with a small field of view is utilized, as it minimizes the number of digital scout images that must be obtained to center the lesion in the aperture of the compression paddle. The skin over the lesion is marked with a felt-tip pen, and this mark is used in positioning the patient for the biopsy procedure. If prone dedicated stereotaxic equipment is utilized, it should be remembered that the lesion may drop closer to the floor than the mark on the skin (which is made in the sitting position) because of the force of gravity on the dependent breast.

Positioning the Patient

Excellent patient positioning is essential in achieving good results with stereotaxic biopsy and requires close cooperation of radiologist, technologist, and patient. If stereotaxic biopsy is performed with the patient prone, the patient is usually positioned with her head turned away from the radiologist's working area and with both arms down at her sides. A thin pillow can be placed between the table and the patient's abdomen. Lesions close to the chest wall may be particularly challenging; placing the patient's arm and shoulder into the opening through which the breast protrudes may be helpful in some cases. For lesions in areas of the breast surrounded by insufficient tissue to allow the excursion of the needle, rolling the breast, adjusting the position of the tube, or selecting a different approach may be necessary.

The breast must be immobilized for stereotaxic biopsy. Compression is applied at the time of the scout film and maintained throughout the biopsy procedure. The amount of compression should be adequate to prevent motion and obtain high-quality images, but must be tolerable for the patient.

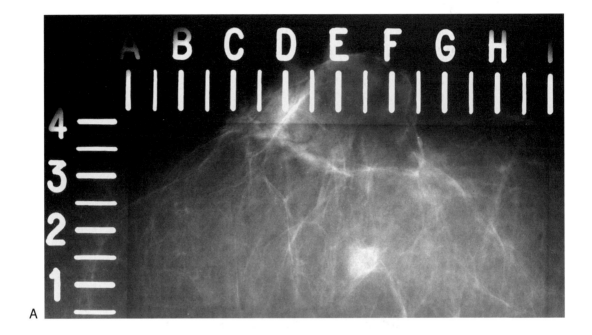

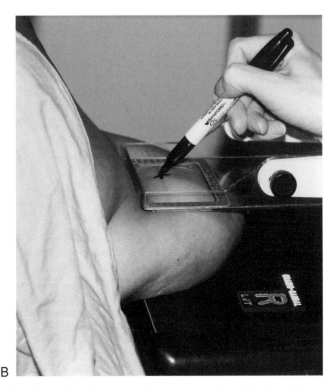

Fig. 9-1. (A) Prebiopsy localizing film obtained with breast positioned in the alpha-numeric grid. The lesion is an irregular nodule, which was new from prior mammograms. **(B)** The skin overlying the lesion is marked with a felt-tip pen.

Scout Film and Stereotaxic Images

An attempt should be made to center the lesion on the horizontal or x axis on the scout image, so that the lesion remains within the field of view for the angled stereotaxic images (Fig. 9-2). If the lesion is not centered on the x axis, adjustments should be made in positioning and a repeat scout image obtained. Centering the lesion on the vertical or y axis is not essential. After the scout image is obtained, it is helpful to mark the skin with a felt-tip pen at the location of the corners of the aperture of the compression plate, so that any patient motion will be easily recognized. The two 15-degree oblique stereotaxic images may then be performed.

Targeting the Lesion

Successful targeting requires selecting the same point in the lesion on both stereotaxic images (Fig. 9-3). For masses, the initial target is generally the central point of the mass. For calcifications, the same calcification must be selected on both images—either a calcification centrally located within the cluster or one particularly distinctive in its morphology—so that it can be reliably identified on the two stereotaxic images. Recent improvements in software assist the operator in targeting the same point on the two stereotaxic images and allow the operator to select multiple targets based on one set of stereotaxic views (Fig. 9-3).

The location of the first target is communicated to the stereotaxic equipment via a hand-held computer "mouse." For film-screen systems, the location of the target and two reference points on each image are indicated on films placed on a digitizer. For digital systems in which the images are displayed on a monitor, the mouse controls a cursor, which is placed at the target point on both images. The computer mechanism then indicates the x, y, and z coordinates of the lesion. These coordinates can be transmitted from the viewing monitor to the biopsy unit by pressing a button.

Assessing the Adequacy of Breast Thickness

The excursion or "throw" of the automated biopsy gun is equal to the distance that the needle will travel in the tissue when the gun is fired. For "long-throw" guns, this distance is equal to 2.2 to 2.3 cm. If the needle were placed at the center of the lesion, then most of the sampling would be from beyond the lesion. To sample tissue from the lesion, the needle is pulled back before firing. The pull-back distance should bring the needle tip to the leading edge of the lesion. The appropriate pull-back distance, therefore, is approximately half the size of the lesion. For a 1-cm lesion, for example, the pull-back distance should be approximately 5 mm.

The stroke margin is defined as the distance that remains between the needle tip and the back breast support after the gun is fired. This number must be greater than zero to safely perform the core biopsy. If biopsy is performed with a negative stroke margin, the needle will strike the back breast support. This outcome should be avoided for at least two reasons. First, the skin surface opposite the site of needle placement has not been anesthetized, and striking it would be painful for the patient. Second, the force of impact could cause damage to the stereotaxic equipment or to the needle, causing it to bend or even to break inside the breast. Therefore, adequacy of stroke margin should always be checked before performing the biopsy. This number is indicated on a display on currently available equipment. Some equipment has a safety mechanism that emits an audible signal if the needle has been placed at a depth that will cause a negative stroke margin.

The adequacy of breast thickness should be assessed before making the scalpel incision for needle placement (Fig. 9-4). The stroke margin (SM) can be calculated by the following formula:

$$SM = T - (z - P) - E$$

where T is the thickness of the compressed breast, z is the depth of the lesion as determined by the computer, P is the pull-back distance, and E is the excursion of the gun. Alternatively, SM also can be determined before needle placement by bringing the needle to a depth of zero (outside the skin surface), checking the SM, and subtracting the prefire position of the needle $(z - P)$ from the SM indicated. If the calculated SM is negative, the breast should be repositioned before needle placement.

Preparing the Breast

The skin within the aperture of the compression plate is cleansed with iodine soap, such as Betadine. A

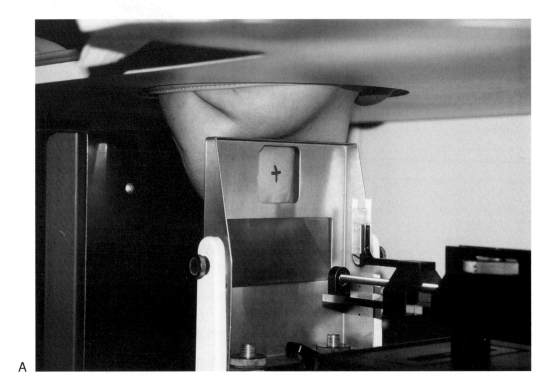

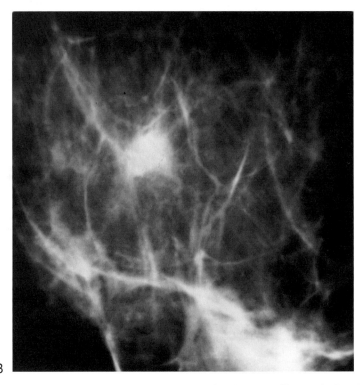

Fig. 9-2. (A) The patient is positioned in the stereotaxic unit for the scout film, with the skin mark centered in the aperture of the compression plate. **(B)** The scout film demonstrates the lesion in good position, approximately in the midline on the horizontal or x axis.

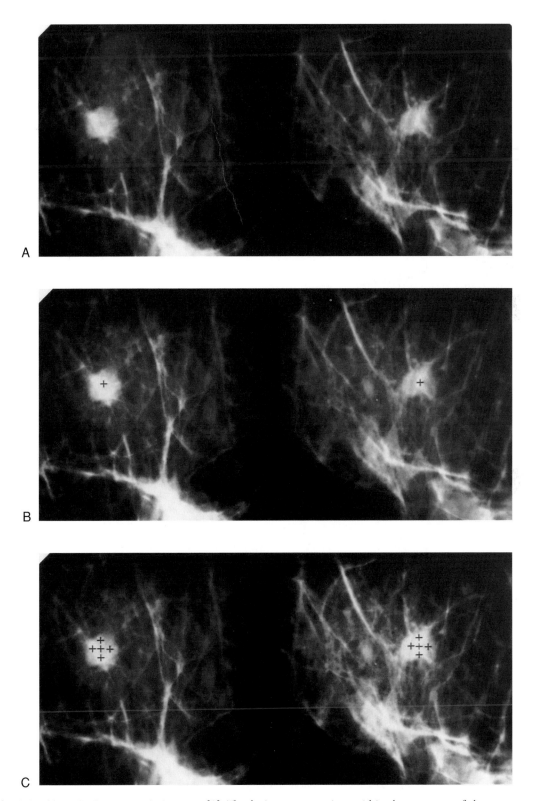

Fig. 9-3. "Targeting" stereotaxic images. **(A)** The lesion must project within the aperture of the compression plate on both images. **(B)** The central point within the lesion has been identified on both views. **(C)** Some units are equipped with software that allows the radiologist to obtain coordinates on multiple targets within the lesion from one set of stereotaxic images.

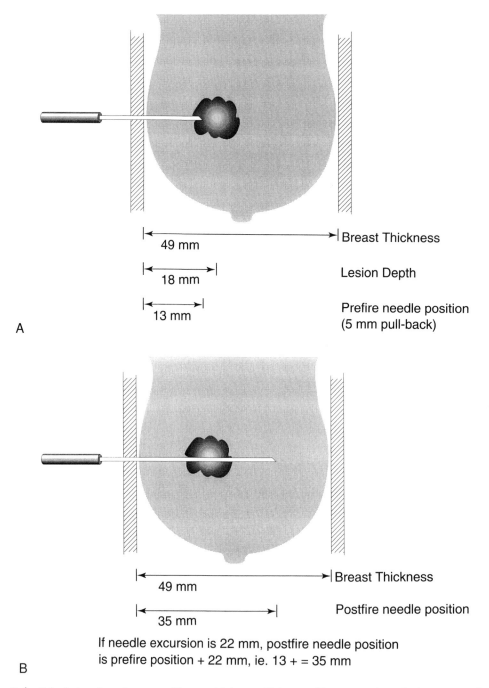

Fig. 9-4. Calculating the adequacy of breast thickness. This case illustrates a 1-cm lesion centered 18-mm deep to the skin surface. The thickness of compressed breast parenchyma is 49 mm. **(A)** Prefire needle position, with pull-back distance of 5 mm. **(B)** Postfire needle position. The stroke margin is equal to the thickness of the compressed breast parenchyma minus the postfire needle position (i.e., 49–35 = 14 mm. This positive number indicates that the thickness of breast parenchyma is adequate to perform the biopsy.

sterile needle holder is positioned between the gun holder and the skin of the breast. The biopsy needle is placed in the spring-loaded automated gun. It is helpful to explain to the patient that when the biopsy is performed, she will hear a loud clicking noise. It is also useful to fire the gun in the air before needle placement, so that the patient knows what to expect. It may also diminish patient anxiety if she does not see the gun and needle during the procedure. This approach minimizes the chance that the patient will jump in surprise or fear when the biopsy is being performed. The gun is then mounted into position and tightened in place with a side screw; it is important to ensure that the gun is fully advanced in its holder. For some equipment, the operator enters the data regarding needle length on a variety of needles and then selects the needle to be used at the outset of the procedure. For other equipment, each new needle utilized must be "zeroed": the tip of the needle is lined up with the upper, outer edge of the aperture of the compression plate, and the appropriate button is pressed on the stereotaxic unit.

The needle is then set to the appropriate x and y coordinates. One sets the x and y values to those given by the computer; if the coordinates have been transmitted, this should bring the "differential" for x and y each to zero. Motorized stands are available that will automatically set the x and y coordinates to those determined by the stereotaxic unit at the time the coordinates are transmitted; if such equipment is not available, the x and y coordinates can be adjusted manually. The needle is then brought to the skin surface, indicating the site of skin incision.

Local anesthesia is given with a 25-gauge hypodermic needle. A subcutaneous wheal is raised and deep anesthesia is given, up to 2 to 3 cc. Patients may experience less discomfort during anesthetic injection if the deep anesthesia is administered first. In our practice, lidocaine (1 percent) is utilized as an anesthetic agent. The addition of epinephrine (1:200,000; 5 μg/ml) can approximately double the duration of anesthesia, but is contraindicated in patients for whom adrenergic stimulation is undesirable.[23]

A small linear scalpel incision is made to break up subcutaneous fibrous tissue, which may hamper the excursion of the biopsy needle. For a round mass, a vertical incision may be preferable because it parallels the direction in which patients tend to move. For calcifications, one can choose the direction of scalpel incision according to the geometric distribution of calcium in the breast parenchyma. For example, if the calcifications line up along the horizontal axis, a horizontal incision may be more useful.

Placing the Needle

After the scalpel incision is made, the needle is placed to the desired depth (Fig. 9-5). Two options are available for depth of needle placement at this step. First, one may place the needle to the depth ("z") indicated by the computer and then obtain prefire stereotaxic images. The needle is then pulled back the appropriate distance immediately before firing. Alternatively, one may place the needle to the depth of z minus the pull-back distance before obtaining the stereotaxic images. With this approach, even if the target is a tiny microcalcification, the needle will be proximal to it and, therefore, should not obscure it. Either approach is acceptable, as long as the radiologist performing the biopsy knows which option was chosen and interprets the prefire images accordingly.

Prefire Images

Two stereotaxic "prefire" images are obtained with the needle in place before tissue sampling (Fig. 9-6). These films allow the radiologist to determine whether the targeting has been accurate. If the needle was placed to a depth equal to "z minus the pull-back," the needle tip should be projected over the leading edge of the lesion on both views. If the needle was placed to the "z" given by the computer, the needle tip should be directly superimposed on the center of the lesion on both prefire stereotaxic images. The needle should then be "pulled back" the appropriate distance before firing.

Errors in targeting may occur on one or more of the x, y, or z axes (Fig. 9-7). X-axis error results in the needle being displaced to the right or the left of the desired location (as determined when one is looking directly at the aperture of the compression plate) on both stereotaxic images. Y-axis error results in the needle tip being displaced either cephalad or caudad to the desired location on the two stereotaxic images. Z-axis error results in the needle tip being either too deep or superficial to the desired location on both stereotaxic images. Needle position must be precisely accurate on both stereotaxic images before firing. If

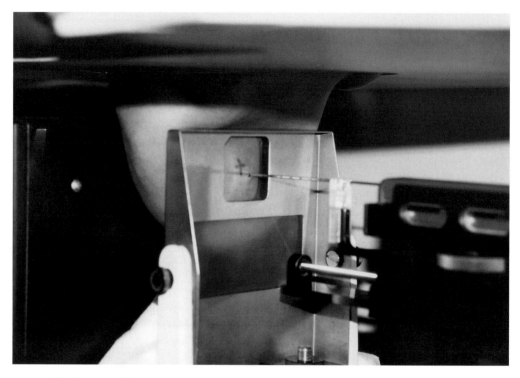

Fig. 9-5. Needle placement for stereotaxic core biopsy with patient in prone position. Notice that the skin mark, which was made with the patient sitting, does not precisely correspond to the needle entry site.

positioning is incorrect on either view, the lesion may not be sampled. It is also important to always remember that although the needle tip may appear well positioned on one of the two stereo views, the image on which the needle is more poorly positioned is the more accurate indicator of its true position.

If the needle is not in the correct position on the prefire images, the radiologist has two options. One option is to utilize the location of the needle tip with respect to the target on the prefire images to estimate the necessary correction; the needle is then removed and repositioned as needed. This approach requires considerable experience. The second option is to "retarget" (i.e., obtain another set of coordinates). This approach usually can be achieved utilizing the prefire stereotaxic images with the needle in place. If the needle tip obscures the desired target, however, the needle should be removed and a new set of "targeting" stereotaxic images obtained. The needle is then placed in the breast in accordance with the new coordinates. Accurate positioning should then be confirmed with a new set of prefire stereotaxic images. When the needle is repositioned within the breast, it is advan-

tageous to remove the needle tip from the area of the lesion, usually to a site where it is just under the skin, and then reintroduce it to the newly calculated position. If the needle positioning is adjusted without removing it from the area of the lesion, the lesion can move its position when the needle is moved to its new coordinates.

Biopsy (First Pass) and Postfire Images

After the needle is accurately positioned to the prefire location, the patient is told that the biopsy will now be performed and that she will hear the noise that has been previously demonstrated for her. The gun is fired and two stereotaxic "postfire" images are obtained (Fig. 9-8). The needle should be observed to traverse through the center of the lesion on these images. Regardless of needle location on the postfire images, the sample obtained is removed and processed as discussed below.

If the postfire images do not confirm that the lesion has been sampled, one may either estimate the necessary correction to needle placement based on the location of the needle tip relative to the target on the post-

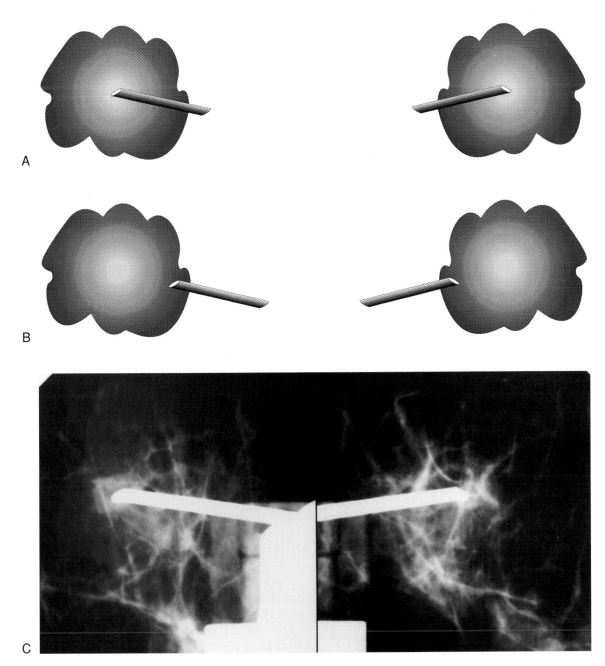

Fig. 9-6. Accurate positioning on "prefire" stereotaxic images. **(A)** Diagram. Needle has been placed to a depth of "z." Needle tip overlies the center of the lesion on both views. **(B)** Diagram. Needle has been placed to a depth of "z minus pull-back." Needle tip is projected over the leading edge of the lesion on both views. **(C)** Case example. Needle has been placed to "z minus pull-back." Needle tip overlies leading edge of irregular nodule on both views.

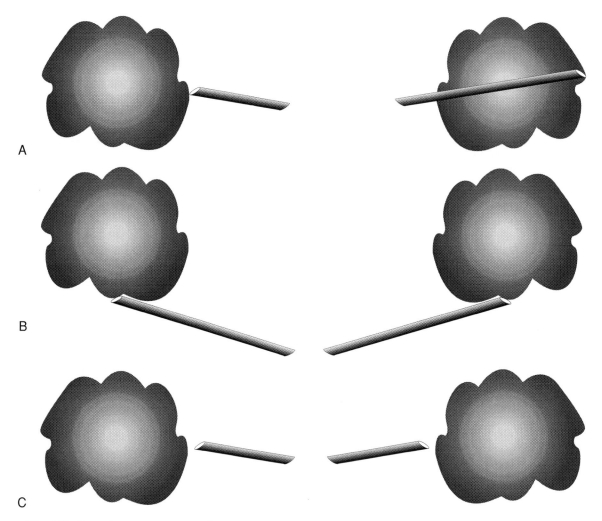

Fig. 9-7. Errors in targeting on "prefire" stereotaxic images. **(A)** X axis error: needle tip is projected to the right of desired location on both views. **(B)** Y axis error: needle tip is projected inferior to desired location on both views. **(C)** Z axis error: needle tip is proximal to desired location on both views.

fire images, or one may "retarget." A second set of prefire and postfire images should be obtained with the second pass if the images from the first pass failed to document that the needle traversed the lesion.

Removing the Specimen

The core must be extracted from the biopsy needle carefully. It is helpful to use the straight edge scalpel with which the skin incision was performed. Sometimes the core adheres to the scalpel; it is often valuable to use a sterile 25-gauge needle, attached to a syringe filled with sterile saline, to help flush the

core off the cutting needle. For masses, cores are then placed in the appropriate preservative as specified by the cooperating pathology laboratory, such as 10 percent neutral buffered formalin. For calcifications, cores are placed on microscope slides for specimen radiography.[27] The biopsy needle and those instruments that touch it should not touch the formalin until the last specimen has been obtained, because the needle will be put back into the patient for subsequent cores, and the formalin can cause tissue damage. After the last biopsy specimen has been obtained, the needle should be swirled in the preservative to remove any tissue that may adhere to it.

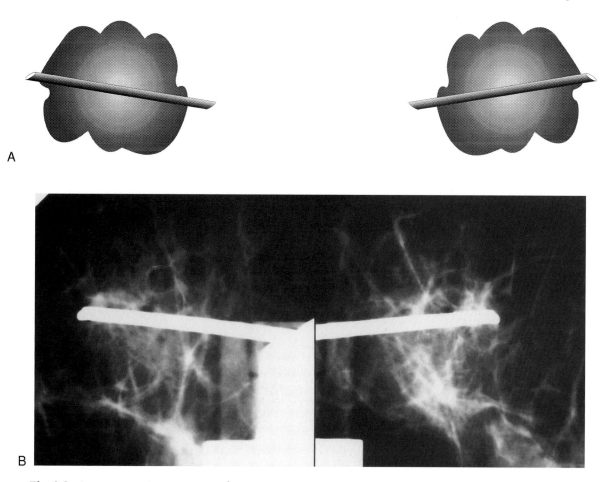

Fig. 9-8. Accurate positioning on "postfire" stereotaxic images. Needle traverses through the center of the lesion on both views. **(A)** Diagram. **(B)** Case example: histopathologic analysis revealed infiltrating ductal carcinoma.

Specimen Radiography

Specimen radiography is an essential component of stereotaxic core biopsy performed for calcifications.[27,28] Immediately after each core is extracted, it is placed on a conventional microscope slide and moistened with normal saline. Slides are serially numbered, and a corresponding lead numeral is positioned adjacent to each slide before it is radiographed. Cores are radiographed using magnification ($\times$1.5) without compression at initial settings of kVp = 23 and mAs = 20 (Fig. 9-9). Specimen radiographs are reviewed during the procedure to determine whether calcifications have been sampled (Fig. 9-10).

I routinely send two separate labeled specimen containers to the pathology laboratory, one containing the cores for which specimen radiography

revealed calcium and one containing the cores for which specimen radiography did not demonstrate calcium. This protocol is helpful to the pathologist because if calcifications are not identified in the initial histopathologic analysis, deeper sections may be obtained from the cores containing radiographically evident calcium. The likelihood that a histopathologic diagnosis will be made for a particular core is 81 percent if calcium is seen at specimen radiography of that core and 38 percent if calcium is not identified.[27]

Subsequent Cores

Subsequent cores usually can be obtained through the same linear scalpel incision made at the outset of the procedure. The new x and y coordinates are set with the needle tip at the skin surface, and then

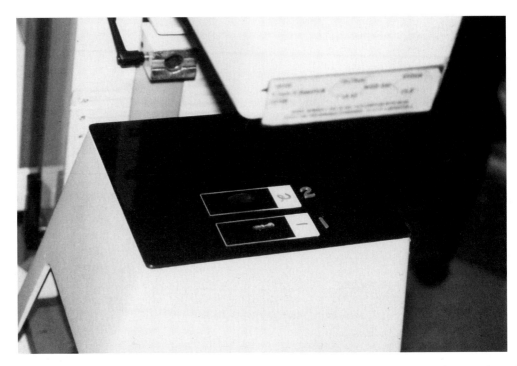

Fig. 9-9. Radiography of core biopsy specimens is performed to determine whether calcifications have been sampled. Microscope slides are placed from left to right on the magnification stand and radiographed without compression at initial settings of kVp = 23 and mAs = 20.

either the needle shaft or the skin can be moved using sterile technique to the position required to guide the needle tip into the incision.

The location of subsequent cores can be determined in one of two ways. One may use the initial target coordinates, as well as lesion size and morphology, to decide the location of subsequent passes, as discussed below. Alternatively, recent software upgrades allow the operator to obtain coordinates for multiple regions of interest using one set of stereotaxic images at the time of initial lesion targeting.

Five core biopsy specimens are usually obtained for masses (Fig. 9-11).[29] The initial biopsy site is the center of the lesion, and subsequent cores are obtained from the 12, 3, 6, and 9 o'clock positions of the lesion without additional imaging. The distance of the subsequent passes from the initial pass varies with lesion size. For large lesions, one may move farther from the central point, but for small lesions, a smaller distance may be needed to stay within the lesion.

For calcifications, a minimum of five core biopsy specimens are obtained, but frequently more are necessary (Fig. 9-11).[13,29] Parker[14] recommends obtaining 10 or more cores for calcifications. The ini-

tial core is taken either from the central point or from a particularly distinctive calcification; subsequent cores are taken either from the 12, 3, 6, and 9 o'clock positions or according to the geographic distribution of calcium in the breast parenchyma. If specimen radiography reveals little or no calcium in the first few cores, the lesion should be retargeted and additional cores obtained. The biopsy is continued until calcium is identified at specimen radiography or until the cores appear to be composed of predominantly hemorrhagic material, which usually occurs within 10 or 12 cores.[29] Ideally, one would like to observe calcium in radiographs of multiple specimens to maximize the likelihood that the core biopsy material is representative and diagnostic.

Postbiopsy

After the procedure, compression is held for approximately 5 minutes. It may be useful to use an ice pack while applying pressure to help achieve hemostasis. The wound is then cleansed with alcohol or peroxide, and a sterile bandage is applied. The patient is told she can shower in the morning, but not to take a bath or

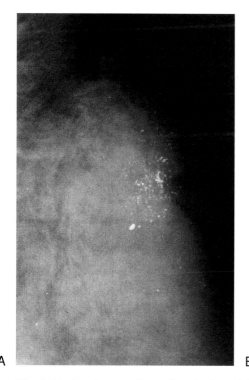
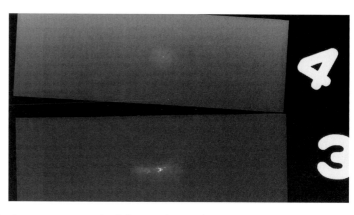

Fig. 9-10. Specimen radiography of microcalcifications: case example. **(A)** Coned magnified view of a cluster of pleomorphic microcalcifications in a dense breast. **(B)** Radiography of stereotaxic core biopsy specimens revealed calcifications. Histopathologic analysis of core biopsy material yielded intraductal carcinoma, comedo type.

completely immerse the breast in water for 2 days and to avoid strenuous activity for a few days. Instructions are given to her verbally and in writing. She is also given the phone number of the radiologist performing the biopsy and told when she will be contacted with the results. If she does not hear from the radiologist, she is instructed to call. She is also asked to call if she is concerned about bleeding or any other complication. It is not necessary to obtain a mammogram immediately after stereotaxic core biopsy. The postbiopsy mammogram is inferior to specimen radiography for documenting that calcifications have been sampled. [29a] The postbiopsy mammogram is also compromised in its ability to serve as a new baseline by the frequent presence of minor postbiopsy changes such as air and mild hematoma.[29a]

Stereotaxic Fine Needle Aspiration Biopsy

The details of FNAB are discussed elsewhere in this book; however, a few points are made here. Many of the preliminary steps of stereotaxic FNAB, including selecting approach, preliminary grid-localizing film,

positioning, and targeting the lesion, are identical to those steps for stereotaxic core biopsy; but there are a few differences. The appropriate needle must be selected or "zeroed" and attached to a 10-cc syringe. Connecting tubing may be used to attach the needle to the syringe if desired. A sterile needle holder specific for fine needle aspiration is utilized. The skin is cleansed and anesthetized, but a scalpel incision is not necessary.

Just as in stereotaxic core biopsy, the needle for stereotaxic FNAB is placed to the calculated x, y, and z coordinates and prebiopsy stereotaxic images obtained. Unlike in core biopsy, however, for which the needle must be "pulled back" 5 to 7 mm from the calculated z depth before biopsy, the needle for FNAB must be placed to the distal aspect of the lesion. For a 1-cm lesion, for example, the needle is placed 5 mm beyond the central point.

Sampling for FNAB is performed by making multiple excursions of the needle while applying suction to the syringe. The amplitude of the excursions usually should be greater than 1 cm. It is helpful to rotate the needle between excursions and to make slight (5- to

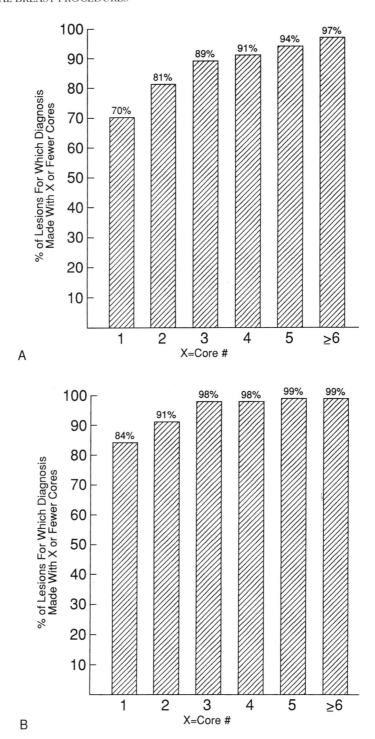

Fig. 9-11. Diagnostic yield for sequential core biopsy specimens for (**A**) all lesions (n = 145), (**B**) masses (n = 92). *(Figure continues.)*

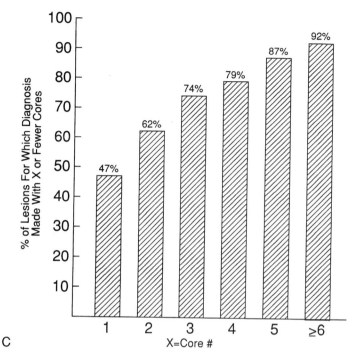

Fig. 9-11. *(Continued).* (**C**) calcifications without mass (n = 53). Note that obtaining five core biopsy specimens resulted in a histopathologic diagnosis in 99 percent of masses but in only 87 percent of calcifications without mass. (From Liberman et al,[29] with permission.)

10-degree) changes in the angle of the needle during sampling.[30] After sampling is complete, suction is released while the needle tip is within the lesion and the needle is withdrawn.

Material is then analyzed on site or processed to be sent to the cytology laboratory. The syringe is disconnected from the needle, filled with air, and reattached to the needle. The cellular material is then expelled onto slides. Placing the slides back-to-back in 95 percent alcohol is one accepted approach to specimen processing for FNAB. Alternatively, smears can be sprayed with fixative. The specimens should be processed in accordance with the preferences of the interpreting pathology laboratory. Having a cytologist or cytopathologist on site at the time of the procedure may decrease the rate of inadequate samples and is likely to yield the best results.

As with core biopsy, multiple passes are desirable, with three to five being standard in the absence of an on-site cytopathologist. After biopsy, the area is compressed, cleansed, and covered with sterile gauze or a bandage.

Reviewing the Pathology Report and Notifying Patient and Physician

It is the radiologist's responsibility to review the pathology reports on all cases for which he or she performed the biopsy. The pathology report must be interpreted in conjunction with the imaging studies, and the pathology and imaging results should be concordant before the pathology results are accepted as appropriate. If inadequate tissue is obtained or if there is discordance between imaging and pathology results, further evaluation is needed, with either repeat stereotaxic biopsy or surgical biopsy. Surgical excision should be recommended for all cases in which atypical ductal hyperplasia is noted because of the high prevalence of carcinoma in these lesions at surgery.[13,31] Surgical excision is also indicated if stereotaxic biopsy histology suggests the possibility of certain lesions that are best assessed with wider tissue sampling, such as phyllodes tumors, or lesions that have a high association with carcinoma, such as radial scars.

In my practice, if a specific benign diagnosis is made at stereotaxic core biopsy that is concordant with the imaging characteristics, the patient is referred for mammography in 1 year. If carcinoma is identified, the patient consults her surgeon, discusses treatment options, and (in most cases) proceeds to have a therapeutic surgical procedure. It should be remembered that a core biopsy diagnosis of ductal carcinoma in situ (DCIS) does not exclude the presence of invasive carcinoma at surgery. Of lesions yielding DCIS at stereotaxic core biopsy, the likelihood that invasive cancer will be found at surgery is approximately 20 percent.[13,32]

The radiologist must notify the referring physician of the results of the stereotaxic biopsy. The decision regarding who notifies the patient should be made by the radiologist and physician. In our practice, the radiologist notifies both physician and patient of all results and gives specific recommendations for future management. It is important to be sensitive in communicating these results to the patient, particularly if carcinoma is detected. The final, written biopsy procedure report from the radiologist should include the histopathology results and management recommendations, and should document to whom the results were communicated.

Follow-up

The radiologist should attempt to obtain follow-up data on all patients who undergo stereotaxic biopsy. It is helpful to develop a mechanism for retrieving this information when a stereotaxic biopsy program is being established. For patients who undergo surgery after stereotaxic biopsy, the radiologist should correlate the surgical histopathology results with the needle biopsy findings. The radiologist must have this information to assess the accuracy of stereotaxic biopsy in his or her own practice.

CONCLUSION

Recent work has demonstrated that the use of stereotaxic core biopsy in the diagnosis of indeterminate or suspicious mammographically detected lesions of the breast can decrease the cost of diagnosis by more than 50 percent.[33] Stereotaxic biopsy can be performed quickly,[18] resulting in less time lost from work or home activities, and complications are rare.[25] At a time when health care policy and reimbursement decisions are influenced by cost considerations, increased utilization of stereotaxic biopsy may decrease the cost of diagnosis of mammographically detected cancers. Meticulous attention to technique may allow maximal realization of the benefits of the stereotaxic biopsy procedure.

REFERENCES

1. Bolmgren J, Jacobson B, Nordenstrom B. Stereotaxic instrument for needle biopsy of the mamma. Am J Roentgenol 1977; 129:121–125.
2. Svane G, Silfversward C. Stereotaxic needle biopsy of nonpalpable breast lesions: cytologic and histopathologic findings. Acta Radiol Diagn 1983; 24:283–288.
3. Dowlatshahi K, Jokich PM, Schmidt R, et al. Cytologic diagnosis of occult breast lesions using stereotaxic needle aspiration. Arch Surg 1987; 122:1343–1346.
4. Dowlatshahi K, Gent HJ, Schmidt R, et al. Nonpalpable breast tumors: diagnosis with stereotaxic localization and fine-needle aspiration. Radiology 1989; 170:427–433.
5. Parker SH, Lovin JD, Jobe WE, et al. Stereotactic breast biopsy with a biopsy gun. Radiology 1990; 176:741–747.
6. Fajardo LL, Davis JR, Wiens JL, Trego DC. Mammography-guided stereotactic fine-needle aspiration cytology of nonpalpable breast lesions: prospective comparison with surgical biopsy results. Am J Roentgenol 1990; 155:977–981.
7. Parker SH, Lovin JD, Jobe WE, et al. Nonpalpable breast lesions: stereotactic automated large-core biopsies. Radiology 1991; 180:403–407.
8. Dowlatshahi K, Yaremko ML, Kluskens LF, Jokich PM. Nonpalpable breast lesions: findings of stereotaxic needle-core biopsy and fine-needle aspiration cytology. Radiology 1991; 181:745–750.
9. Mitnick JS, Vazquez MF, Roses DF, et al. Stereotaxic localization for fine-needle aspiration breast biopsy. Arch Surg 1991; 126:1137–1140.
10. Dronkers DJ. Stereotaxic core biopsy of breast lesions. Radiology 1992; 183:631–634.
11. Elvecrog EL, Lechner MC, Nelson MT. Nonpalpable breast lesions: correlation of stereotaxic large-core needle biopsy and surgical biopsy results. Radiology 1993; 188:453–455.
12. Gisvold JJ, Goellner JR, Grant CS, et al. Breast biopsy: a comparative study of stereotaxically guided core and excisional techniques. Am J Roentgenol 1994; 162: 815–820.

13. Jackman RJ, Nowels KW, Shepard MJ, et al. Stereotaxic large-core needle biopsy of 450 nonpalpable breast lesions with surgical correlation in lesions with cancer or atypical hyperplasia. Radiology 1994; 193:91–95.

14. Parker SH. Stereotactic large core breast biopsy. In Parker SH, Jobe WE (eds). Percutaneous Breast Biopsy. Raven Press, New York, 1993; 61–79.

15. Hendrick RE, Parker SH. Principles of stereotactic mammography and quality assurance. In Parker SH, Jobe WE (eds). Percutaneous Breast Biopsy. Raven Press, New York, 1993; 49–59.

16. Caines JS, McPhee MD, Konock GP, Wright BA. Stereotaxic needle core biopsy of breast lesions using a regular mammographic table with an adaptable stereotaxic device. Am J Roentgenol 1994; 163:317–321.

17. Dershaw DD, Fleishman RC, Liberman L. Use of digital mammography in needle localization procedures. Am J Roentgenol 1993; 161:559–562.

18. Parker SH, Dennis MA, Jobe WE, Hendrick RE. Clinical efficacy of digital stereotaxic mammography. Radiology 1993; 189 (Suppl):326.

19. Sickles EA. Periodic mammographic follow-up of probably benign lesions: results in 3,184 consecutive cases. Radiology 1991; 179:463–468.

20. Sickles EA, Parker SH. Appropriate role of core breast biopsy in the management of probably benign lesions. Radiology 1993; 188:315.

21. Logan-Young WW, Janus JA, Destounis SV, Hoffman NY. Appropriate role of core breast biopsy in the management of probably benign lesions. Radiology 1994; 190:313.

22. Sickles EA, Parker SH. Reply. Radiology 1994; 190:313–314.

23. Ritchie JM, Greene NM. Local anesthetics. In Gilman GG, Rall TW, Nies AS, Taylor P (eds). Goodman and Gilman's The Pharmacological Basis of Therapeutics. 8th Ed. Pergamon Press, Elmsford, NY, 1990; 311–331.

24. Page CP, Bohnen JMA, Fletcher JR, et al. Antimicrobial prophylaxis for surgical wounds: guidelines for clinical care. Arch Surg 1993; 128:79–88.

25. Parker SH, Burbank F, Jackman RJ, et al. Percutaneous large-core breast biopsy: a multi-institutional study. Radiology 1994; 193: 359–364.

26. Kaye MD, Vicinanza-Adami CA, Sullivan ML. Mammographic findings after stereotaxic biopsy of the breast performed with large-core needles. Radiology 1994; 192:149–151.

27. Liberman L, Evans WP, Dershaw DD, et al. Radiography of microcalcifications in stereotaxic mammary core biopsy specimens. Radiology 1994; 190:223–225.

28. Meyer JE, Lester SC, Frenna TH, White FV. Occult breast calcifications sampled with large-core biopsy: confirmation with radiography of the specimen. Radiology 1993; 188:581–582.

29. Liberman L, Dershaw DD, Rosen PP, et al. Stereotaxic 14-gauge breast biopsy: how many core biopsy specimens are needed? Radiology 1994; 192:793–795.

29a. Hann LE, Liberman L, Dershaw DD, et al. Mammography immediately after sterotaxic breast biopsy: is it necessary? Am J Roentgenol 1995; 165:59–62.

30. Fajardo LL. Stereotactic fine-needle aspiration breast biopsy. In Parker SH, Jobe WE (eds). Percutaneous Breast Biopsy. Raven Press, New York, 1993; 89–94.

31. Liberman L, Cohen MA, Dershaw DD, et al. Atypical ductal hyperplasia diagnosed at stereotaxic core biopsy of breast lesions: an indication for surgical biopsy. Am J Roentgenol 1995; 164:1111–1113.

32. Liberman L, Dershaw DD, Rosen PP, et al. Stereotaxic core biopsy of breast carcinoma: accuracy at predicting invasion. Radiology 1995; 194:379–381.

33. Liberman L, Fahs MC, Dershaw DD, et al. Impact of stereotaxic core biopsy on cost of diagnosis. Radiology 1995; 195:633–637.

10

INTERVENTIONAL BREAST ULTRASONOGRAPHY

Ellen B. Mendelson

Of the imaging techniques available for guiding interventional procedures, ultrasound is the most direct.[1-4] Compared with stereotaxic mammographic guidance, even with a digital assist to speed the procedure, sonographic guidance of fine needle aspiration of fluid-filled and solid masses, core biopsy, and presurgical localization is rapidly accomplished. Using free-hand technique, the positioning, adjustment, and final placement of the needle tip can be observed in real time.

One of the most important applications of breast sonography is to guide interventional procedures. These procedures include cyst aspiration and abscess drainages, fine needle and large core needle biopsy of solid lesions, and presurgical localizations.

X-ray and magnetic resonance (MR)-guided percutaneous procedures and open surgical biopsies, as well as a comparison of the indications, merits, and drawbacks of each, are discussed elsewhere in this text. This chapter focuses on sonographically guided percutaneous procedures, patient preparation, equipment selection, procedural performance, and suggestions for successful accomplishment.

PATIENT PREPARATION, EQUIPMENT, AND TECHNIQUES FOR ULTRASOUND-GUIDED PROCEDURES

The initial steps are the same for all of the procedures, as are the mechanics of free-hand, ultrasound-guided needle passage.

Preparing the Patient and the Equipment

Informed consent is obtained from the patient before any of these procedures is performed. The procedure and its purpose should be described and the complications mentioned; the patient should indicate her understanding of what will follow (Table 10-1).

Once the patient assumes the appropriate position for the procedure, the breast should be cleansed with alcohol and Betadine (Purdue Frederick Company, Norwalk, Connecticut). The probe should be disinfected with alcohol, although probes should not be soaked in alcohol. If manufacturers suggest that alcohol not be used at all, a solution such as Cidex (Johnson and Johnson, Arlington, Texas) can be painted on the transducer face, the probe housing, and the portion of the cord entering the probe housing. Although some radiologists prefer to cover the probe with a sterile plastic sheath or wrap, it is not necessary to sheath a transducer as long as it is carefully prepared as above.[5] Sheathing of the probe may degrade the image and impair manual control of the breast and instrument, making the procedure more difficult to accomplish. The operator and any assistant must wear gloves at all times, primarily for their own protection.

If it is known before scanning that an aspiration will be performed, it will save time if patient consent is obtained, the patient's breast is cleansed, and the operator's and assistant's hands are gloved in advance. Sterile gel should be used as a coupling agent for scanning the breast. During the procedure

Table 10-1. Complications of Ultrasound-Guided Interventional Procedures

When obtaining consent from patients, pertinent medical history should be elicited so that potential complications can be discussed and, in some cases, avoided.

Bleeding

Obtain a history of anticoagulation, chronic aspirin use, or blood dyscrasias; discuss brief interruption of medication such as warfarin sodium (Coumadin) with referring physicians. Laboratory assays may be helpful in individual cases.

Infection

A potential complication that is uncommon with breast interventional procedures but should be mentioned. Antibiotic prophylaxis for patients with rheumatic heart disease or mitral valve prolapse has not been deemed necessary.

Localized pain

Tenderness and ecchymosis are common. Ordinarily, they are self-limited, but it is important that the patient will expect discoloration of the skin of the breast and some discomfort that may be treated with aspirin or Tylenol. Immediately after the procedure, we provide an ice pack to the patient.

Pneumothorax

Use the technique of needle entry from the short axis of the transducer where the needle passes through the acoustic beam along the long axis of the probe. Avoid steep approaches in the medial aspect of the breast near the chest wall where the pleura is only a short distance from the aspirating needle.

itself, however, alcohol or Betadine can be used as a coupling agent, remoistening the skin as necessary.

It is helpful to have all of the required materials available in the ultrasound room or on a cart that can be brought in without notice. Procedures are most easily incorporated into busy schedules if the staff and equipment are in perpetual states of readiness.

Techniques of Percutaneous Needle Passage

There is no single correct method for performing these procedures, and free-hand sonographically directed needle placement utilizes the same principles for fine needle aspiration of cysts and solid lesions, presurgical localization, and core biopsy.

Selection of a technique to guide the procedure should reflect the location, the nature of the lesion, and the particular procedure being performed. A deeply situated small mass in a large, fatty breast may be aspirated, biopsied, or localized more easily using mammographic (fenestrated compression plate or stereotaxic) guidance than with ultrasound.

For safe, ultrasound-guided aspiration of lesions near the chest wall or adjacent to the implant shell of an augmented breast, the needle shaft must be visualized during the entire procedure (Fig. 10-1). Using this technique with needle entry from the short axis of the transducer, the mass can be positioned anywhere along the length of the transducer. The more horizontal the plane of entry, the better the needle shaft will be visualized; it is important that the needle tip not veer from the narrow acoustic beam. If the needle angles to the right or to the left rather than remaining midplane, the tip will no longer be seen. If the lesion is deep, it is best to position it at some distance from the entry point of the needle so that a more horizontal approach can be used. Superficial lesions can be positioned near the end of the transducer, and the needle directed more vertically into the lesion.

If the lesion is far from the chest wall and the breast is stabilized, presurgical localizations and some cyst aspirations can be performed with a more steeply vertical approach from the midportion of the long axis of the transducer (Fig. 10-2). This route of entry may offer the shortest distance to the lesion, which the surgeon may prefer. In general, however, use of this second technique is limited, and the approach diagrammed in Figure 10-1 should be selected for its safety and the visualization of the needle shaft during the entire procedure.

Linear transducers of 7.0 MHz or greater frequency are best for free-hand procedures. Needle guides are offered with some transducers, particularly those of arrays other than linear, but I have not found these guides, which support the needle and allow for variable angles of entry, to diminish the difficulty of the procedure or to increase its accuracy.

Difficulties with needle tip visualization have led to the development of coated, pitted, or scored needle tips to increase the echogenicity. An additional factor affecting needle visualization is the needle gauge, with larger caliber needles more easily seen. An inge-

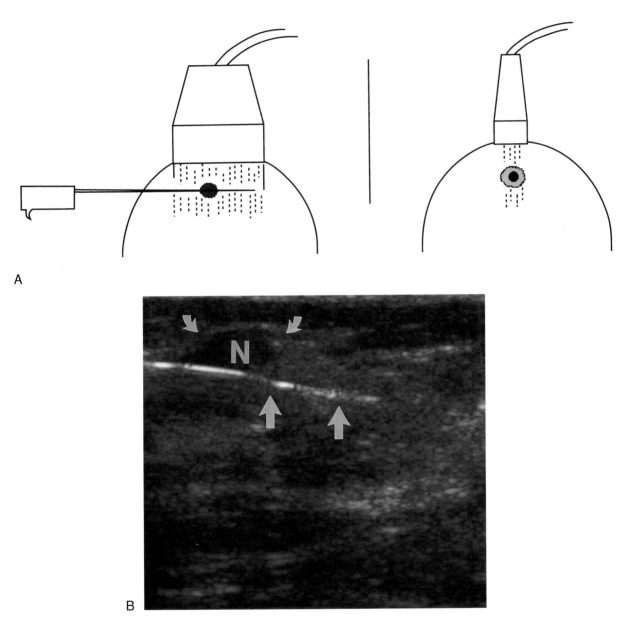

Fig. 10-1. (A) Technique for free-hand ultrasound-guided needle procedures: short axis entry. The needle shaft will be visualized if the needle path remains aligned with the acoustic beam. The more horizontal the entry, the more completely the needle shaft and tip will be seen. This is the technique of choice for safe needle passage in approaching lesions near the chest wall or the shell of a silicone implant and for core biopsies with spring-activated devices that propel the needle forward. **(B)** Horizontal needle path and core biopsy of complex mass. Complex cystic mass (*curved arrows*) contains mural nodule (N) within it. Note the shallow angle of the needle after firing. The collecting area of the needle (*straight arrows*) samples the solid nodule, an intracystic papillary carcinoma.

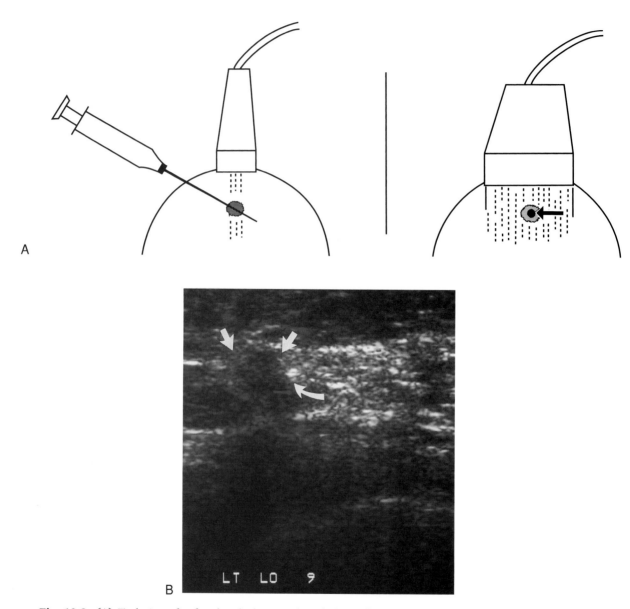

A

B

Fig. 10-2. (A) Technique for free-hand ultrasound-guided needle procedures: long axis entry. Needle entry from the long axis of the transducer with the lesion centrally placed in the image is useful for some cyst aspirations and presurgical localizations of relatively superficial masses. The needle crosses the acoustic beam, and only a portion of the needle shaft is seen (*arrow*). Tip location cannot be confirmed. This method is not desirable for guiding large needle core biopsy or for approaching lesions near the chest wall. **(B)** Presurgical localization of small hypoechoic cancer (*arrows*) using this approach. The needle shaft is not seen. The echogenic dot (*curved arrow*) represents the portion of the needle passing through the acoustic beam. This approach may provide the shortest distance from the skin to the lesion. After ultrasound-guided needle localization, craniocaudal and lateral mammograms should be obtained for use in the operating room.

nious device is the transponder, which allows a signal to be emitted by the transducer as it traverses the tissue. The signal is brightly echogenic and helps to visualize the course and ultimate destination of the needle.[6] A similar effect is created by causing microvibrations of the needle during its passage through the breast tissue. With color flow imaging, the needle will be seen without difficulty. Motion makes the needle path more readily identifiable, and the moving needle itself will be seen as an artifact.[5]

Personnel

These procedures can be staffed in several ways. One person may hold the probe and aspirate, or assistants may be helpful in holding the probe. If an assistant scans, the performer of the procedure has both hands available. To stabilize the probe, it should be held near the base. If even pressure is exerted on the lesion, it is less likely to roll out of the field. As the lesion is kept in view, one hand can be placed against the breast to help stabilize the lesion. The needle can then be guided into the mass. One of the most important requirements for success is immobilizing the lesion under the transducer. A second is placement of the probe to allow monitoring of the direction of needle entry and passage with respect to the anticipated path of the acoustic beam.

SPECIFIC PROCEDURES

For all ultrasound-guided procedures, the same techniques can be used. The following sections describe the specific techniques of cyst aspiration, fine needle aspiration biopsy (FNAB) of solid lesions, core biopsy, and presurgical localization.

Cyst Aspiration

Breast cysts are common in the perimenopausal years and may persist or develop in postmenopausal women receiving hormone replacement therapy. Breast sonography can allow the diagnosis of a simple cyst if four criteria are fulfilled: (1) oval or round shape, (2) anechogenicity, (3) sharply defined margins, particularly the posterior wall, and (4) posterior acoustic enhancement.[7,8]

Indications for Sonographically Guided Aspiration[8]

The following are indications for sonographically guided aspiration of cystic lesions:

1. Masses that do not fulfill the sonographic criteria for simple cysts (Fig. 10-3)
   a. Internal echoes, particularly if all of the technical factors such as gain and power settings and focal zone placement have been adjusted and there are other cysts in the breast that appear anechoic
   b. Irregular or thickened margins
   c. Lack of posterior acoustic enhancement despite positional and pressure maneuvers to change the relationship between the transducer and the breast (if the mass is directly above the pectoral muscle, enhancement is difficult to demonstrate)
2. Nonpalpable cysts that are symptomatic in causing local tenderness
3. Palpable cysts in which it might be important to document evacuation or any residual fluid
4. Palpable or nonpalpable cysts in which imaging guidance would help avoid complications (e.g., with breast implants or cysts near chest wall)

Technique

The area of the cyst should be fixed manually so that the needle will penetrate the wall of the lesion rather than push it out of the scan plane. Choice of needles, the aspirating apparatus, use of assistants, and other details may vary. A small-caliber needle may be selected initially, and if the cyst contents are of low viscosity, evacuation of the cyst will be rapid and successful. If a tough, fibrous rind encases the cyst, the needle may be deflected; if the cyst contains viscous material, the lesion may empty slowly or not at all. A stiffer, larger bore needle will then be required to enter thick-walled lesions that resist needle penetration. If the first attempt to aspirate with a 21-gauge needle is unsuccessful, the second attempt is made with an 18-gauge needle. Alternatively, 19- or 18-gauge needles may be used at the outset. To avoid a second needle stick, I routinely use an 18-gauge needle for cyst aspiration.

Attempts should be made to avoid passing the needle through the very sensitive areola. The areolar skin

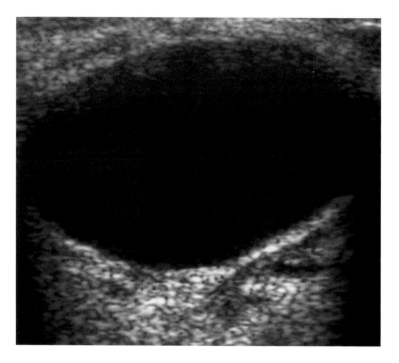

Fig. 10-3. Simple cyst. Four criteria must be fulfilled for the diagnosis of simple cyst: anecho-genicity, round or oval shape, sharp margins, and posterior acoustic enhancement. Near field artifactual echoes may be present anteriorly in a cyst, but the deeper portion should be echo free and the posterior margin sharp.

can be stretched and pulled out of the way, allowing access to the cyst. If it is necessary to pass the needle through or near the areola, lidocaine is injected with a tuberculin syringe. The local anesthesia can be introduced from a site adjacent to the areola and burrowed under it to raise a wheal. In most other instances, although we offer lidocaine to patients, cyst aspirations are performed without local anesthesia.

For cyst aspiration, contents of a cyst of 2 to 3 cm or less can be accommodated with a 10-ml syringe. If the cyst is very large, use of a 20-ml syringe and connecting tubing is efficient in cyst evacuation. For smaller cysts, a hypodermic needle and syringe, aspirating gun, or vacutainer type of device works well. For small hands in tight places, negative pressure can be maintained with less exertion using an aspirating gun for cyst and fine needle aspiration than with a syringe alone. Several lightweight aspirating guns are currently available.

I aspirate during continuous scanning, not removing the probe from the site until the procedure is completed. Sonograms are obtained before and immediately after the procedure, usually with the needle still in

place. They are labeled "preasp" and "postasp," the location given by clock notation; the initials of the physician who performed the procedure also are included. The postprocedural sonogram may be useful for comparison in follow-up studies of the area of aspiration. A postaspiration mammogram (Fig. 10-4) is obtained in lateral position or whatever view shows best the concordance of mammographic and sonographic abnormalities.

Cyst Fluid

Practice patterns vary with regard to disposition of cyst fluid. Some facilities submit all cyst aspirates for cytologic evaluation, but many radiologists and surgeons discard yellow or serous aspirates and greenish fluids suggestive of fibrocystic change. Any bloody or other unusual cyst aspirate must be analyzed cytologically. If the aspirate is purulent, microbiologic study (culture and sensitivity) should be requested in addition to cytology. Lesions should be evacuated and drainage catheters may be placed in abscesses if aspiration is incomplete and a significant residuum is present.

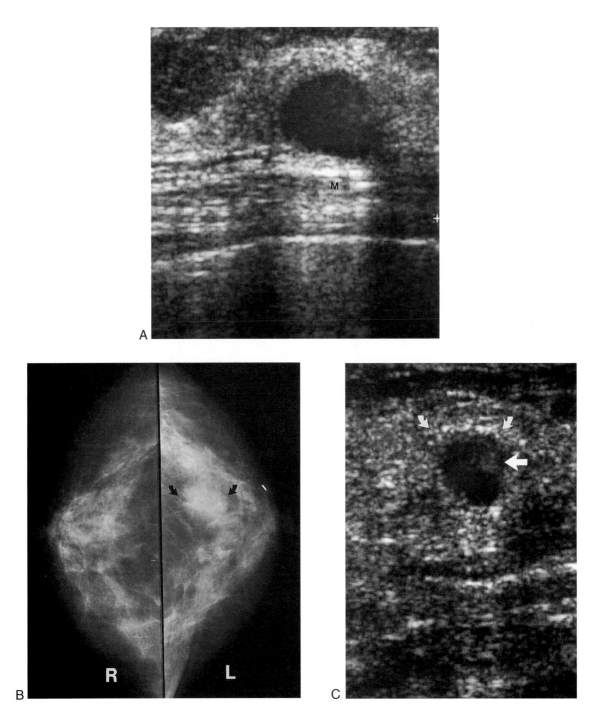

Fig. 10-4. Cystic masses. Cystic or complex masses not fulfilling the criteria for a simple cyst should be aspirated. Occasionally, it may be difficult to differentiate solid and fluid-filled masses, and aspiration should be the first step. If fluid is not obtained, the needle that has already been placed may be used to obtain cellular material for cytologic analysis. **(A)** Abscess. Sonography in an area of tenderness reveals a hypoechoic lesion with unevenly dispersed internal echoes and posterior acoustic enhancement just anterior to the pectoral muscle (M). Aspiration yielded pus. **(B & C)** Abscess. **(B)** Craniocaudal mammographic view shows small oval soft tissue density (*curved arrows*) whose margins are obscured by surrounding parenchyma. Small metallic marker denotes area of focal pain. **(C)** Mass is predominantly anechoic but contains echogenic clump anteriorly (*straight arrow*). There is marginal irregularity except posteriorly, and an echogenic rim is also present (*curved arrows*) seen with abscesses and some carcinomas. Ultrasound-guided aspiration yielded pus. Abscesses are most commonly caused by staphylococci. *(Figure continues.)*

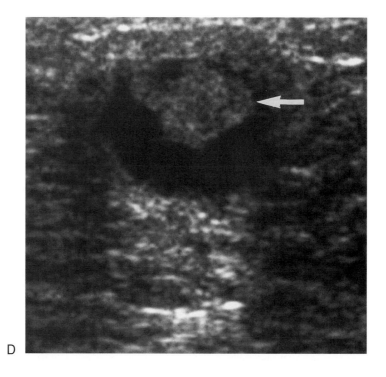

D

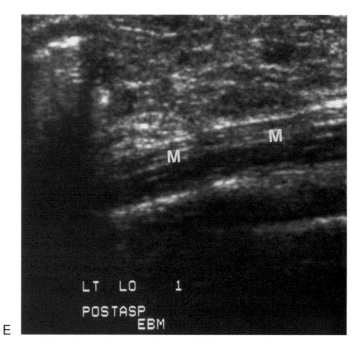

E

Fig. 10-4. *(Continued).* **(D)** Galactocele. Ultrasonography of a nontender palpable mass in a lactating woman shows echogenic material clumped anteriorly (*arrow*) within an otherwise simple-appearing cyst (smooth borders, oval shape, posterior acoustic enhancement). A whitish-yellow oily fluid representing milk product and butterfat was obtained from the mass on aspiration. **(E)** Postaspiration sonogram shows complete evacuation of galactocele, with only fat lobules seen anterior to the pectoral muscle (M). *(Figure continues.)*

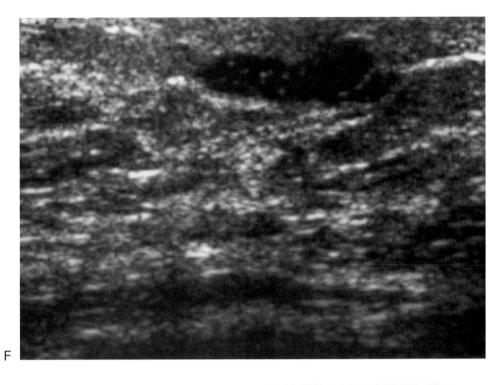

F

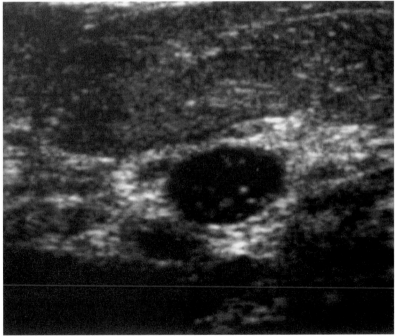

G

Fig. 10-4. *(Continued).* **(F)** Dilated, obstructed duct. Elongated tubular structure, with scattered low-level anterior echoes extending toward the areolar complex. Inspissated debris was aspirated from this obstructed duct. **(G)** Hemorrhagic cyst. Ultrasound-guided aspiration of the cyst with scattered low-level echoes yielded congealed hemorrhagic material. No malignant or atypical cells were identified. One week earlier, however, the patient's gynecologist had attempted aspiration of the mass by palpation.

Pneumocystography is more fully discussed in Chapter 3. It has been proposed as a means of sclerosing the cyst and preventing reaccumulation of fluid.[9,10] The physiologic explanation is somewhat obscure, and there has been no subsequent documentation of the effectiveness of pneumocystography in preventing reaccumulation of cysts in a large group of women. Careful sonography should obviate the need for delineation of cyst walls by pneumocystography. A mural excrescence should be evident sonographically, using high-resolution, high-frequency transducers. In some cases, an important justification for performing pneumocystography is to place a marker within the breast so that if localization or aspiration is desired at a later time, the air can be used as such a marker.

Pneumocystography is performed by injection of slightly less air than the amount of fluid obtained.[9] The syringe with fluid is removed while the needle remains in the breast, and another syringe preset to deliver the appropriate amount of air is attached. After the air has been introduced, orthogonal craniocaudal and 90-degree lateral views are obtained. The air injected may remain for a period of time. The pneumocystogram can be used as a map from which measurements can be made if a return to the area is desired at some time after the procedure.

Sampling Solid Lesions: Fine Needle Aspiration Biopsy and Large Needle Core Biopsy

Indications and recommendations for FNAB and core biopsy are the following:

1. A mass thought to be malignant to confirm the diagnosis so that a one-stage surgical procedure can be performed
2. More than one mass where the possibility for multifocal (one quadrant) or multicentric (two or more different quadrants) malignant disease exists, again to facilitate treatment planning
3. Ambivalence about follow-up versus excision, and the patient, radiologist, and referring physician seek greater confidence in foregoing surgical removal of a probably benign lesion such as a fibroadenoma
4. A hypoechoic structure whose features are not that of a simple cyst—although many of these masses are cysts, others are fibroadenomas, papillomas, or circumscribed carcinomas.[2,8] If a hypoechoic mass is

new, particularly if it is solitary, it should be sampled rather than followed.
5. Indeterminate masses with greater likelihood of benign than malignant etiology (BIRADS, Category 3)[11]

Fine Needle Aspiration Biopsy

Despite using an 18-gauge needle and visualizing the needle tip in the appropriate location, if no fluid is obtained from a mass that might have represented a complex cyst, a slide should be made of the needle contents for cytopathologic evaluation. If the cytologic preparation is inadequate or the interpretation not definitive, a new solid mass should undergo core biopsy or be excised surgically.

Sonographically guided fine needle aspiration will be successful when all of these following requirements are met:

1. Familiarity with ultrasonographic appearances of many breast lesions
2. Experience with using ultrasound to guide the procedure
3. Confirmation that the needle has entered the periphery, the center, or any other area of the lesion desired
4. Effective aspiration technique to obtain sufficient cellular material unadulterated by blood
5. Immediate preparation of slides according to the preferences of the cytopathologist. If a cytopathologist or cytotechnologist is present, sufficiency of the samples can be confirmed before concluding the procedure
6. Experience of the cytopathologist in evaluating breast lesions should at least match that of the radiologist doing the procedure

Techniques

Using one of the two free-hand approaches described earlier, short excursions into the lesion should be made under sonographic guidance with a 21- to 23-gauge needle and syringe with negative pressure applied. These brief but numerous up-and-down excursions should allow material from the mass to enter the needle. If blood is seen, the pass should be concluded, and the slide made. In withdrawing the needle, gentle release of negative pressure will allow the syringe plunger to return to a neutral position, and the aspirated material will not be drawn into the syringe itself. To prepare the slide, the syringe should be disengaged from the needle and air drawn in. The syringe then should be reattached to the needle, and the contents of the needle expelled onto a slide and fixed as directed by the cytopathologist. For some stains, immediate fixation is desirable. Some cytopathologists ask for the slides to be air dried and prepared with Diff-Quik solution.

A modification of technique involves the use of an aspirating gun. Several models are available, some of them quite light and easy to manipulate. Many of these guns use 10-ml syringes, are easy to manipulate, and allow even the smallest hand to exert good negative pressure for collection of the aspirate.

Another method involves use of a 23- or 25-gauge needle, without a syringe. The same short excursions are made into the lesion. By capillary action, cells will enter the needle.[1] A syringe containing a few milliliters of air should be attached to the needle and the contents of the needle expelled onto a slide, prepared as described earlier.

Still another technique is to use a coaxial needle apparatus with placement of a 19-gauge outer cannula at the edge of the lesion. A smaller (21-gauge) aspirating needle is then introduced. With use of a coaxial system, only one puncture is required.

Fine needle aspiration cytology performed by an experienced mammographer or sonologist and interpreted by seasoned cytopathologists should provide reliable diagnoses of malignancy with no false-positive results. Frequently, a direct or inferential identification of a fibroadenoma can be made through "naked nuclei" or epithelial cells consistent with a fibroadenoma.[12] More difficult are the diagnoses of fibrosis, fat necrosis, and infiltrating lobular carcinoma where tumor cells travel single file within the stroma and do not ordinarily have a spherical pattern of growth.

Core Biopsy

Large Core Needle Biopsy

Large core needle biopsy has become an important breast diagnostic procedure in the last several years. Because of the variability of cytopathologic expertise in the United States, with insufficient samples reported in up to 25 percent of cases in some series, nonsurgical tissue sampling to provide cores for histologic analysis has grown popular.[9] Both stereotaxic mammography and ultrasound have proved to be accurate in guiding needle placement, and each has advantages. The reliability of large core needle sampling as a substitute for

surgical biopsy has been asserted by Parker and others.[13-16] Core biopsies are performed with spring-activated guns (several manufacturers including Bard, Bip, and Manan) using a 14-gauge needle. This needle provides tissue samples of greater tissue cohesiveness for histopathologic analysis than breast specimens obtained with 18-gauge needles.[17] Pathologic interpretations have been definitive in most cases.[3]

Uses for core biopsy are the same as those for FNAB as listed earlier, but with the addition of widespread or multifocal microcalcifications and groupings of indeterminate calcifications. Ordinarily, calcifications are sampled using stereotaxic mammographic guidance. Core biopsies are recommended if the biopsy of more than one region would affect and determine treatment options. For example, if two widely separated areas show ductal carcinoma in situ, modified radical mastectomy might be selected in preference to breast conservation. The location of the lesion, its visibility with ultrasound, and the radiologist's comfort level and experience with the various techniques will determine the approach selected. For some stereotaxic equipment, the posterior breast near the chest wall is inaccessible, and the conical retroareolar area may not provide enough tissue tension within the window of the stereotaxic compression plate for a good biopsy. In these instances, a mass or occasionally widespread microcalcifications, some of which may be demonstrated sonographically, are appropriate targets for sonographically guided core biopsy. When sampling microcalcifications with core biopsy, specimen radiographs of these cores provide important evidence that calcifications are within the tissue cores.

Sonographically guided procedures have several advantages. They provide choice in positioning of the patient; a supine or supine-oblique position may be more comfortable for the patient than the prone or seated positions required for stereotaxic mammographic core biopsies. Real-time observation of needle passage and its entry into the lesion cannot be achieved with stereotaxic methods, and ultrasound procedures may be accomplished more quickly than stereotactically guided biopsies, even with a digital assist.

As with other needle procedures, patients should be told about complications that can occur with core biopsy. These include bleeding, bruising and tenderness, and as with any needle procedure, pneumothorax and infection. Infection is unreported, and pneumothorax is rare. I have observed that bleeding with the supine-oblique positioning is less common than with the prone position used for mammographic stereotaxic aspirations. With stereotaxic biopsies, the dependent breast may become engorged with venous blood, and a fair amount of free bleeding may occur during the procedure. I have not had a problem with postprocedural hemostasis, in general, and have seen the formation of only a few small hematomas. A case of needle track seeding of a mucinous carcinoma after core biopsy has been reported.[18] Viability of cells is unknown, and spread of disease or carcinomatosis after percutaneous biopsy of the lungs and abdominal organs, which has been performed for many years, has not been an issue.

Technique for Ultrasound-Guided Core Biopsy

The general technique is diagrammed in Fig. 10-1 and described earlier. For greatest safety, the needle shaft should be visualized completely as it remains within the narrow acoustic beam. The danger of penetration of the chest wall or an implant is minimized, and the performer of the procedure has greater control with this technique.

Approximately 2 ml of 1 percent lidocaine is used. A lidocaine or saline channel from the skin to the lesion can be used to indicate the angle of entry of the 14-gauge needle and to ease the initial 14-gauge needle passage, sometimes associated with some resistance during the first pass. A small amount of sodium bicarbonate mixed with the lidocaine may prevent the burning sensation associated with the local anesthetic.[3] A skin wheal is made with a 25-gauge needle. Most of the nerve endings in the breast are in the skin and superficial tissues, and even when using a 14-gauge needle, it is unnecessary to infiltrate more deeply. Frequently with sonography, the delivery of lidocaine can be observed. A small mass can be obscured or displaced by the lidocaine, although lidocaine injected posterior to a deep lesion can elevate it so that the 14-gauge needle can be directed more superficially with less risk of penetrating the chest wall. Care should be taken to try to eliminate all air from the lidocaine before it is injected, as it can obscure the targeted lesion and the needle tract.

A small skin nick is made, wide enough so that a 14-gauge needle can be passed easily without its catching at the skin. One skin nick is ordinarily all that is necessary. The needle can be directed under sonographic guidance to sample areas of the mass. Coaxial systems for use with ultrasound-guided core biopsies have been developed.[19] Here the sheath

remains in place while the inner needle is reinserted and manipulated to sample various areas of the mass.

Under sonographic visualization of its passage, the needle should be directed toward the lesion. The gun should be fired at a distance from the mass that accounts for the size of the lesion, the location of the sampling area 0.4 cm back from the tip of the needle, the 1.7 cm length of the sampling area, and thrust of the needle when the gun is fired (2.2 to 2.3 cm with the currently preferred "long throw") (Fig. 10-5).[17,20]

Using a syringe with saline to dislodge the specimen or immersion of the needle in a vial or sterile saline, each specimen is placed into a single or separate jars of 10 percent formalin fixative. The core needle should not be placed directly into formalin if the needle is going to be reinserted into the patient. The cores should be inspected, and a "good core" can easily be differentiated from a fatty sample or fragmented specimen. If the abnormality contains calcifications, radiography of the cores will help confirm their presence in the sample.

Working with the pathology department, one can arrive at an appropriate number of passes to yield a definitive diagnosis. In my practice, although I am involved in a study protocol[15] that requires five stereotaxic passes (central and the four quadrants), I make a greater number of passes for microcalcifications, but for ultrasound core biopsies I ordinarily perform three to five passes into different areas of the lesion.

My patients undergoing core biopsy have reported little pain or discomfort during the procedures. The use of local anesthesia effectively blocks pain sensation at the skin, and the extremely rapid propulsion of the needles using the spring-activated guns also may help reduce both discomfort and anxiety.

Several spring-activated guns are available, and these are discussed in detail in Chapter 6. Some important considerations, however, are reviewed here. Some guns are disposable and convenient, but these are more expensive. Permanent guns are similar but are variably modified. The Biopty (Bard) gun requires removal of the needle from the gun to unload the specimen into formalin. The needle must then be resituated within the gun's mechanism, and the gun cocked. This gun has a heavy, tight spring and fast action that obtains good cores of tissue. The Manan gun has a lever rather than a loop type of handle. This gun is efficient to use, and if the handle is pulled back once, the needle is unsheathed, and the specimen can be placed in formalin without removing the needle. A second pull

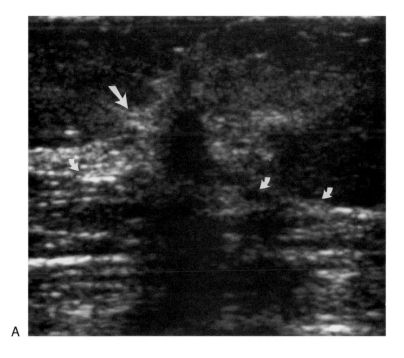

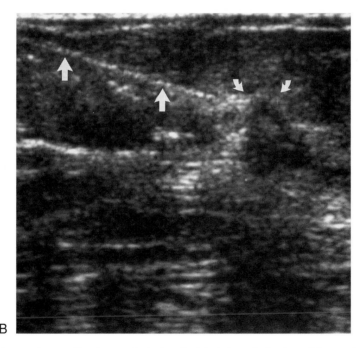

Fig. 10-5. (A) Tubular carcinoma. Poorly marginated, spiculated, irregularly shaped hypoechoic lesion with posterior acoustic attenuation. Note Cooper's ligament (*straight arrow*) being retracted into the surrounding echogenic desmoplastic rind. The tumor is adjacent to the pectoral muscle bundle (*curved arrows*). **(B)** Core biopsy: prefire. On prefire images, the needle tip (*arrows*) is positioned several millimeters away from the mass (*curved arrows*) to allow for the 2.2 cm advance of this long-throw spring-activated sampling device. (*Figure continues.*)

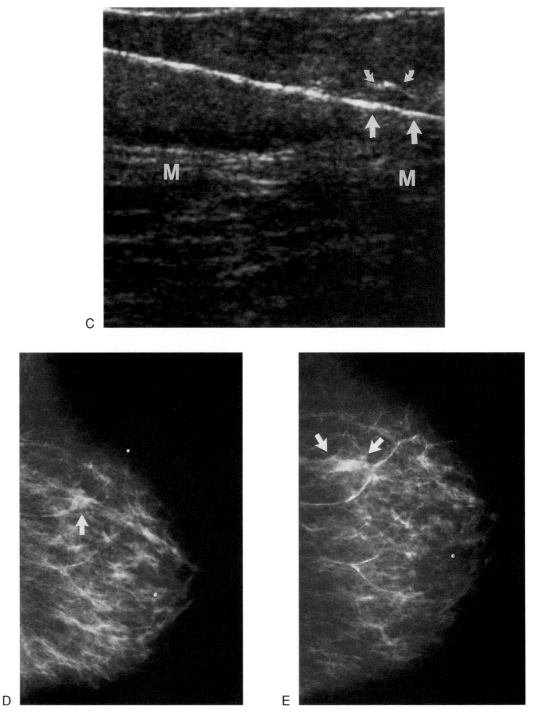

Fig. 10-5. *(Continued).* **(C)** Core biopsy: postfire. A postfire image provides confirmation that the needle shaft has traversed the lesion. The collecting portion of the needle (*arrows*) lies within this mass. Core histology was tubular carcinoma. **(D)** Preprocedure mammogram shows triangular mass (*arrow*). Small metallic pellet on the skin was placed during sonographic evaluation, and a view tangential to the maker was obtained to confirm correspondence of the mammographic and sonographic findings. **(E)** Postprocedure lateral view demonstrates increased soft tissue density and stranding (*arrows*) representing a small amount of bleeding in the area of the triangular density confirming that the biopsied target has been sampled. Note that no large hematoma has formed after the five 14-gauge passes have been made.

up on the lever will resheath the needle, and it is again ready for use. Compared with the Bard, the spring has a slightly looser coil, requiring less force to cock it, but samples have been excellent. A third, the BIP gun, modified recently, is another variation, which is also being developed by other manufacturers for use with similar devices. With this gun, the needle also does not require removal from the apparatus to unload the specimen. The BIP gun also has been adapted for use with coaxial systems.

Review of cytologic or histologic findings is important in assessing the success of procedures and in choosing fine needle or core biopsy. In making this selection, preferences and expertise of the pathologist in the facility must be considered. Malignant masses often prove positive with either technique. For more difficult cytologic diagnoses, including fibrosis, fat necrosis, and infiltrating lobular carcinoma, core biopsy appears to provide better specimens for analysis. Fibroadenomas can be difficult to locate; they are notorious for their evasiveness and can be pushed out of the way by any needle attempting to pierce them. Here, the technique for fine needle and core is to stabilize the lesion by placing a hand on the breast just above the transducer so that the tissue is less likely to move, and to use as little gel or coupling agent as possible.

Presurgical Localization

An important procedure that can be accomplished with sonographic guidance is needle hookwire localization.[4] There are several advantages to using sonographic guidance rather than a fenestrated mammographic plate. The patient is often in supine-oblique or supine position as for surgery, and frequently the approach is that of the shortest distance from the skin to the lesion, which surgeons ordinarily prefer. The approach may or may not be parallel to the chest wall, as is essentially required for the safety in fenestrated plate mammographic localizations. Either the method described in Fig. 10-1—the safest approach when the lesion is near the chest wall, located in the far medial breast or in any other area where the risk of complications is greater— or that shown in Fig. 10-2—which provides probably the shortest distance, can be used.

In general the following lesions are candidates for ultrasound guidance: (1) lesions inaccessible to mammographic fenestrated plate localizations such as high in the axillary tail of the breast or situated far

posteriorly and (2) any mass or other lesion that can be imaged with ultrasound.

The patient need not be supine or in an oblique position; she may be seated or standing if the lesion is best seen and approached in those positions. If the lesion is well circumscribed and hypoechoic and it is possible that it represents an atypical cyst, it is better to remove the hookwire from the needle before it is placed. If fluid emerges from the needle, a syringe can be attached, and the lesion evacuated.

Some needle hookwire assemblies are better suited to afterloading (i.e., insertion of the hookwire after the needle has been placed in the breast). "V" wires are easier to reinsert than curved wires. The curved wire, however, can be put back into the needle. First, it must be loaded through a hypodermic needle, with the straight side going through the beveled end of the needle. Then, the "J" wire must be pulled completely into the hypodermic needle so that the curved end does not protrude. At that point, the hypodermic needle can be piggybacked onto the localization needle into which the wire can be fed.

Once it has been determined that the needle has been placed correctly, the hookwire can be deployed in the tissue. Alternatively, mammographic confirmation of the needle's location can be obtained before hooking the wire.

If the wire is hooked at sonography, my practice is to obtain craniocaudal and lateral mammograms that show the location of the hookwire. Whether or not the lesion has been seen mammographically, surgeons are more accustomed to mammograms than sonograms, and these fully labeled views should be sent to the operating room for use in planning the surgical approach.

Localizations performed with sonographic guidance are accomplished quickly, and if there are scheduling problems, an ultrasound-guided localization can be underway simultaneously with a needle localization in a mammographic room. Combined use of imaging techniques can promote efficient throughput of patients in a breast center.

As with all nonpalpable lesions localized before surgery, a specimen image is essential. A mammographic localization requires a specimen radiograph, and sonography offers the option of obtaining the specimen images with mammography or ultrasound (Fig. 10-6). If sonography is the only technique in which the lesion was seen, a specimen sonogram may be selected. We immerse the specimen in saline, scan

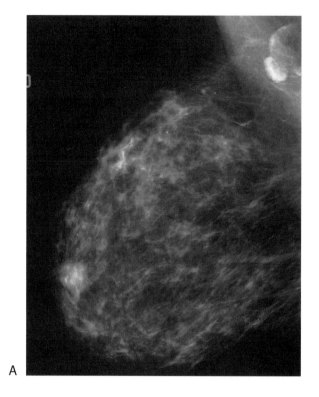

A

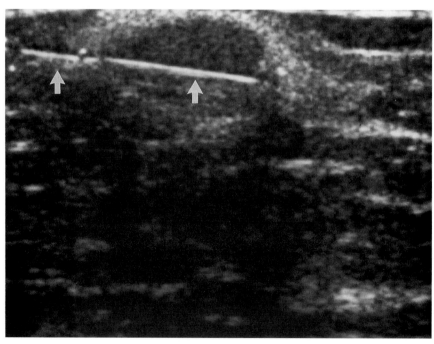

B

Fig. 10-6. Core biopsy: benign appearing mass. **(A)** Lobulated, retroareolar soft tissue density on baseline mammogram, mediolateral oblique view in a 40-year-old woman. Ultrasound showed it to be solid with benign features. The patient requested large core needle biopsy for reassurance that the mass was not malignant. **(B)** The core needle (*arrows*) biopsy provided histology of the hypoechoic oval mass: chronic cystic disease. Interval follow-up studies were elected rather than open surgical excision.

through the saline, and record the image on film. The specimen is then returned to the pathology laboratory.

Even if the lesion were not seen mammographi-cally, a specimen radiograph may be helpful. With the better compression and magnification that is possible for a tissue specimen than in vivo, it is pos-

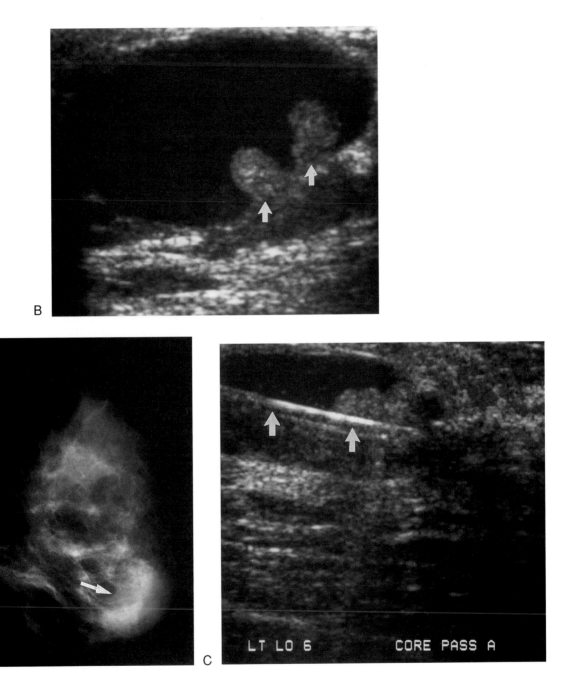

Fig. 10-7. Intracystic papilloma. **(A)** Left mediolateral oblique mammographic projection reveals a large retroareolar soft tissue density (*arrow*) whose posterior margins fade into the surrounding fibroglandular parenchyma. **(B)** With ultrasound a cyst containing hypoechoic papillary projections is seen (*arrows*) along the posterior wall. **(C)** Seen with ultrasound-guided core biopsy, the nodular component can be targeted for sampling. Needle shaft is seen within the mass, and the core sample was identified as an intracystic papilloma.

sible to see an abnormality that was not perceptible on preoperative mammograms.

In any case, both sonographic and mammographic localizations require that a specimen be sent for imaging correlation and the findings reported to the surgeon in the operating room before the incision is closed.

CONCLUSION

Facility with ultrasound-guided breast interventional procedures, as well as familiarity with mammographic, stereotaxic, and computed tomographic-guided procedures allows for flexibility and versatility in selecting among nonsurgical alternatives for breast diagnosis and management (Fig. 10-7). The expected result should be to improve the efficiency and cost-effectiveness of patient care.[21, 22]

ACKNOWLEDGMENT

I greatly appreciate the assistance of Corinne E. Tobin, M.D. in the preparation of this chapter.

REFERENCES

1. Fornage BD, Coan JD, David CL. Ultrasound-guided needle biopsy of the breast and other interventional procedures. Radiol Clinic North Am 1992; 30:167–185
2. Fornage BD. Interventional ultrasound of the breast. In McGahan JP (ed): Interventional Ultrasound. Williams & Wilkins, Baltimore, 1990; 71–83.
3. Parker SH, Lovin JD, Jobe WE, et al. Stereotactic breast biopsy with a biopsy gun. Radiology 1990; 176:141–147.
4. D'Orsi CJ, Mendelson EB. Interventional breast ultrasonography. Semin Ultrasound CT MR 1989; 10:132–138.
5. Reading CC, Charboneau JW. Ultrasound-guided biopsy of the abdomen and pelvis. In Rumack CM, Wilson SR, Charboneau JW (eds): Diagnostic Ultrasound. Mosby-Year Book, St Louis, 1991; 429–442.
6. Winsberg F, Mitty HA, Shapiro RS, Yeh H-C. Use of an acoustic transponder for US visualization of biopsy needles. Radiology 1991; 180:877.
7. Mendelson EB. Ultrasound secures place in breast Ca management. Diagn Imaging 1991; 120–157.
8. Mendelson EB. Breast sonography. In Rumack CM, Wilson SR, Charboneau JW (eds): Diagnostic Ultrasound. Mosby-Year Book, St Louis, 1991; 541–563.
9. Fajardo LL, Jackson VP, Hunter TB. Interventional procedures in diseases of the breast: needle biopsy, pneumocystography, and galactography. Am J Roentgenol 1992; 158:1231–1238.
10. Tabar L, Pentek Z. The diagnostic and therapeutic value of breast cyst puncture and pneumocystography. Radiology 1981; 141:659–663.
11. Kopans DB, D'Orsi C. American College of Radiology Breast Imaging Reporting and Database System, May, 1993.
12. Kline TS, Kline IK. Guides to Clinical Aspiration Biopsy: Breast. Igaku-Shoin, New York, 1989.
13. Parker SH, Burbank F, Jackman RJ. Percutaneous large core biopsy: a multiinstitutional study. Radiology 1994; 193:359–364.
14. Jackman RJ, Nowels KW, Shepard MJ, et al. Stereotaxic large-core needle biopsy of 450 nonpalpable breast lesions with surgical correlation in lesions with cancer or atypical hyperplasia. Radiology 1994:93: 91–95
15. Brenner RJ, Bassett LW, Dershaw DD. Percutaneous core biopsy of the breast: a multisite prospective trial, abstracted. Radiology 1994; 193(P):295.
16. Elvecrog EL, Lechner MC, Nelson MT. Nonpalpable breast lesions: correlation of stereotaxic large-core needle biopsy and surgical biopsy results. Radiology 1993; 188:453–455.
17. Dowlatshahi K, Yaremko ML, Kluskens LF, Jokich PM. Nonpalpable breast lesions: findings of stereotaxic needle-core biopsy and fine-needle aspiration cytology. Radiology 1991; 181:745–750.
18. Harter LP, Curtis JS, Ponto G, Craig PH. Malignant seeding of the needle track during stereotaxic core needle breast biopsy. Radiology 1992; 185:713–714.
19. Kaplan SS, Racenstein MJ, Wong WS, et al. US-guided core biopsy of the breast with a coaxial system. Radiology 1995; 194:573–575
20. Parker SH. When is core biopsy really core? Radiology 1992; 185:641–642.
21. Hendrick RE, Parker SH. Stereotactic imaging. RSNA Syllabus: A Categorical Course in Physics Technical Aspects of Breast Imaging. Oak Brook, IL 1992; 233–243.
22. Lindfors KK, Rosenquist CJ. Needle core biopsy guided with mammography: a study of cost effectiveness. Radiology 1994; 190:217–222.

11

INTERVENTIONAL BREAST MAGNETIC RESONANCE IMAGING

David P. Gorczyca

Magnetic resonance imaging (MRI) has been proposed as a potential imaging modality to evaluate patients with breast diseases. The most promising results are from studies that have used gadolinium enhancement as part of their protocols.[4,1–7] Initial reports suggested that contrast-enhanced MRI of the breast could potentially differentiate benign from malignant tumors based on enhancement patterns. More recent studies, however, have shown an overlap in the enhancement pattern of benign and malignant breast tumors.[3,5,7–9] To add to the problems of diagnosis of breast diseases with MRI, suspicious breast lesions that cannot be identified on any other imaging modality are being detected. MRI of the breast will have a limited clinical role until MR-guided biopsy/localization can be routinely performed to permit determination of the histology of suspicious lesions detected only by contrast-enhanced breast MRI.

MR-guided biopsy and localization in the head and neck have been performed for several years.[9–14] As a result of the research performed on MR-guided biopsy in the head and neck, several MR-compatible needles and localization wires have been made commercially available.[11] The MR-compatible needles and the techniques developed for MR biopsy of the head and neck can be easily adapted to developing MR-guided breast biopsy and localization. Several researchers have published preliminary results using different MR-compatible breast biopsy devices, all showing promising results.[15,16] This chapter emphasizes the design of MR-compatible breast biopsy/localization devices, potential MR techniques, and limitations to MR-guided breast biopsy/localization.

DESIGN OF MR-COMPATIBLE BREAST BIOPSY DEVICES

In designing an MR-compatible breast biopsy device, one could use many approaches. Most of the required features are similar to those required for mammographic-guided breast biopsy or localization. These features include access to the breast, immobilization of the breast, localization of the breast lesion, and confirmation of needle placement. The unique environment of a magnetic field places additional requirements on the MR-compatible device. The material used to manufacture the device must be compatible with a strong magnetic field. It is not surprising, therefore, that plastics are most commonly used to build these devices. Furthermore, the biopsy device and patient must fit comfortably within the relatively small bore of the magnet. Several open interventional magnets are currently being investigated that may lessen the constraints of space and access to the breast placed by using relatively small-bore magnets.

MR-COMPATIBLE BIOPSY NEEDLES AND LOCALIZATION WIRES

Several MR-compatible needles are commercially available. For MR-guided breast fine needle aspirations, 20- or 22-gauge Lufkin needles (E-Z-M, Glen Falls, New York) can be used. These needles contain a high nickel stainless steel alloy and are compatible with the magnetic field. For MR-guided wire localizations, the Homer wire (Homer, NAMIC, Glen Falls, New York) is a J-wire composed of a nitinol alloy. The Homer nitinol alloy wire is MR compatible; however, the needle provided in the Homer breast localization kit creates an unacceptable degree of susceptibility artifacts and is not MR compatible. Therefore, for MR-guided breast localizations, we use an 18-gauge Lufkin needle in combination with the Homer nitinol alloy localization J-wire. MR-compatible core biopsy guns are presently under development.

PATIENT ENROLLMENT AND MRI TECHNIQUES

The following MR protocol is my current approach to MR-guided breast biopsy/localization using a 1.5 T Signa MR imager. In my protocol, a woman can be enrolled only if a breast lesion is identified by mammography, sonography, or clinical breast examination and will subsequently have a biopsy of this lesion. A dedicated contrast-enhanced MRI of the breast is obtained. A dedicated breast coil, bilateral or unilateral, is needed to obtain adequate resolution and signal-to-noise ratio.[17]

The patient lies prone to decrease the respiratory motion artifact. An MR-guided breast biopsy/localization is considered only if additional suspicious lesions are identified on the breast MRI, which are not identified on other imaging modalities. Currently, patients are scheduled on a different day for MR-guided breast biopsy to allow thorough review of the dedicated contrast-enhanced breast MRI and correlate the MR images with the patient's mammogram, ultrasound, and clinical breast examination.

The compression MR-compatible breast biopsy device has two major components, one to comfortably support the prone patient and a second unit that immobilizes one breast by compression plates, allowing good access to the breast for biopsy or localization (Fig. 11-1). Dual, removable, 3-in, general-purpose, phased array surface coils are easily attached to the compression plate to obtain high resolution images. The compression device can be variably positioned about the x-y plane on a Velcro-covered plate, providing approximately 200 degrees of access to either breast. The ability to rotate the compression device on the Velcro platform allows one to choose the most direct and shortest distance to the breast lesion.

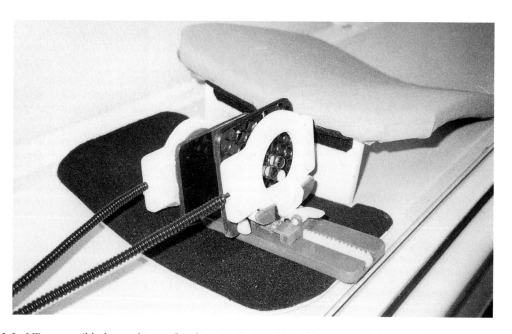

Fig. 11-1. MR-compatible breast biopsy/localization device. The MR-compatible breast biopsy device has two major components, one to support the prone patient, and a second unit that immobilizes one breast by compression plates. Dual removable, 3-in, round, phased array surface coils are easily attached to the compression plates to obtain high resolution images. The compression device can be variably positioned about the x-y plane on a Velcro-covered plate, providing approximately 200 degrees of access to either breast.

The lateral compression plate contains a grid of 13-mm holes that allow needle access to the breast and support a set of gadolinium-doped localizing "bullets." One localizing bullet has a single chamber, a second has one partition, and a third two partitions so that each bullet's position can be identified easily (Figs. 11-2 and 11-3). Each bullet fits snugly into the lateral compression plate grid, allowing accurate identification of the hole closest to the breast lesion.

MR SEQUENCES

We use the following MRI sequences for imaging breast tumors: An axial T_1-weighted scout view is obtained with Fourier-acquired steady-state technique and gradient-recalled acquisition in steady state (FAST GRASS, GE Medical Systems) (repetition time: ms/echo time = 9/3) and a flip angle of 30 degrees. A three-dimensional volume, spoiled gradi-ent-echo (SPGR), (30/5, flip 30 to 60 degree, 128 × 256 matrix; section thickness 1 to 2 mm; fat suppression) is obtained before and after intravenous administration of gadopentate dimeglumine or galacteridol.

The MR sequences used for MR localization of the needle and wire include an axial T_1-weighted spin echo sequence (TR/TE = 400/12, 256 × 256 matrix, 3-mm slices). This is followed by a three-dimensional volume, SPGR, (30/5, flip 30 to 60 degree, 256 × 256 matrix; section thickness 1 to 2 mm). These sequences are repeated to confirm location of additional needles or localization wires. This protocol is only one of many possible approaches.

MR-GUIDED BREAST BIOPSY/ LOCALIZATION PROCEDURE

The technique used for MR-guided breast biopsy is similar to the technique many radiologists use for

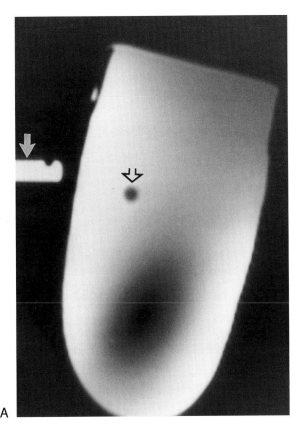
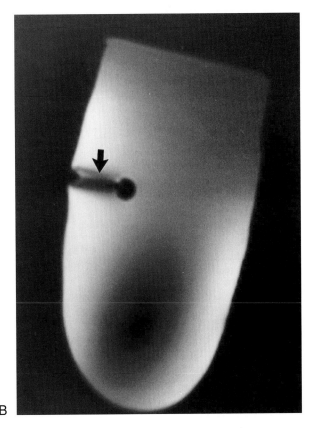

A   B

Fig. 11-2. MR-guided biopsy of breast phantom. **(A)** Localizing bullet (*arrow*) is in good location to biopsy imbedded lesion (*open arrow*) in a breast phantom. **(B)** A 22-gauge Lufkin needle (*arrow*) in good position.

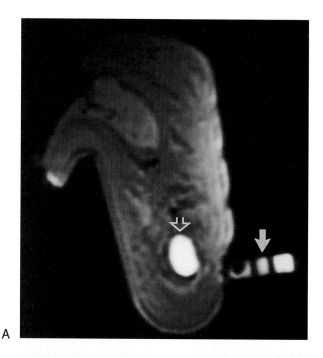

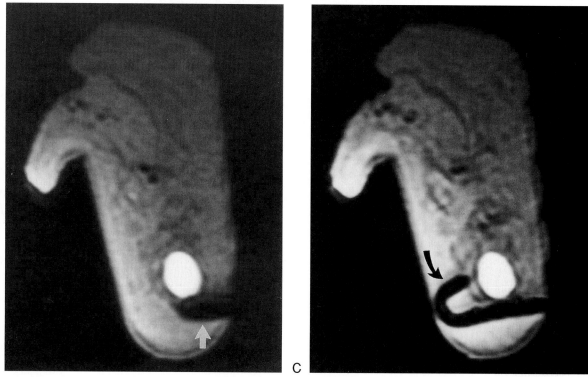

Fig. 11-3. MR-guided localization of cadaveric breast with imbedded gadolinium lesion. **(A)** Localizing bullet (*arrow*, three chambers) in good location to localize breast lesion (*open arrow*). **(B)** An 18-gauge Lufkin needle (*arrow*) in good position before advancing localizer nitinol wire. **(C)** Nitinol wire (*arrow*) in adequate position relative to breast lesion.

computed tomography (CT)-guided biopsies of the chest and abdomen. Before placing the patient on the MR-guided biopsy device, the side compression plate is sterilized either with Betadine or by placing the plate in an autoclave. The patient's breast is then sterilized with Betadine. A high-resolution, three-dimensional volume contrast enhanced MR study is then performed to localize the suspicious lesion. The coordinates of the lesion are recorded on the MR console. The patient is removed from the bore of the magnet, and the localization light on the MR unit is used to position the patient's breast in the correct coordinates. Cross hairs on the localization light mark the zero level on the patient, and a ruler is used to measure the distance of the lesion from the zero position along the z axis. Three different

gadolinium "bullets" are then placed in the three holes closest to the suspicious breast lesion (Figs. 11-2 and 11-3). The patient is imaged to confirm which hole is closest to the breast lesion.

The skin is anesthetized with local anesthetic. An MR-compatible needle is then placed through the hole, and the patient is imaged to confirm the needle position. A fine needle aspiration can be obtained at this point or a localization wire can be placed (Figs. 11-2 to 11-4). The holes in the side compression plate are large enough to allow removal of the compression plate without removing the Lufkin needle/localizing wire combination. The localization wire/needle combination is secured to the breast with gauze and tape. The patient is then transferred to the surgery suite.

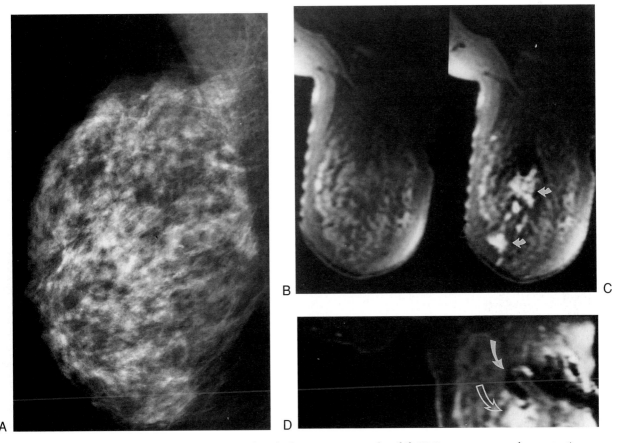

Fig. 11-4. Patient with palpable lesion not identified on mammography. **(A)** MLO mammogram demonstrating dense breast; no breast lesion was identified. **(B)** Pregadolinium and **(C)** postgadolinium image of same breast demonstrating two retroareolar breast lesions (*arrows*). **(D)** Because breast-conserving surgery was scheduled, a localizing nitinol wire (*arrow*) was placed posterior to the lesion (*open arrow*). Infiltrating ductal carcinoma was found at surgery.

LIMITATIONS OF MR-GUIDED BIOPSY

One of the limitations of MR-guided localization is the inability to perform confirmatory specimen images to document that the surgeon actually removed the lesion in question. MRI cannot identify calcifications and some nonenhanced breast lesions as clearly as mammography. A method to reliably confirm that the breast lesion in question was actually removed must be developed for MR localization. One possible solution is to inject a mixture of methylene blue and dilute gadolinium through the needle into the tissues surrounding the breast lesion just before placing the localization wire. If the wire was positioned correctly and the tissues removed accurately, the surgical specimen should demonstrate some increased signal from the gadolinium on a T_1-weighted image. Our limited experience with this technique shows promise. Additional research is necessary, however, to evaluate how gadolinium diffuses in breast tissues.

An alternative solution is to obtain a two-view mammogram of the breast after successful MR-guided localization. Occasionally, one can identify a tissue mass or calcification near the wire localization, which could be used as a marker in a mammographic specimen radiograph to verify that breast tissue near the lesion was surgically removed. Neither of these methods, however, absolutely confirms that the enhancing breast lesion on MRI was successfully removed. Therefore, additional research and methods must be developed to find a reliable method to confirm that the breast lesion was actually biopsied or surgically removed.

SUMMARY

MRI of breast tumors has great potential in selected patients. MRI of the breast occasionally detects lesions not imaged by mammography, especially in women with dense breast tissue (Fig. 11-4). The conspicuity of lesions, especially after the administration of gadolinium, may be superior to what can be identified on two routine mammographic views. The ability to use variable pulse sequences, including tissue suppression techniques, may aid in the detection and characterization of lesions. As a result, MRI could potentially play an important role in differentiating benign and malignant lesions and evaluating the extent of disease, postsurgical breast, and response to chemotherapy or radiation therapy. Until MR-guided breast biopsy/localization is shown to be reliable and widely available, however, MRI of the breast will continue to have a limited clinical role.

ACKNOWLEDGMENT

Peter Sullenberger (Captain Plastic, Santa Ana, CA) built and helped design the MR-compatible breast biopsy/localization device.

REFERENCES

1. Harms SE, Flamig DP, Hesley KL, et al. Fat-suppressed three-dimensional MR imaging of the breast. Radiographics 1993; 13:247–267.
2. Harms SE, Flamig DP, Hesley KL, et al. MR imaging of the breast with rotating delivery of excitation off resonance: clinical experience with pathologic correlation. Radiology 1993; 186:493–501.
3. Heywang SH, Wolf A, Pruss E, et al. MR imaging of the breast with Gd-DTPA: use and limitations. Radiology 1989; 171:95–103.
4. Heywang-Kobrunner SH, Hilbertz T, Beck R, et al. Contrast-material enhanced MRI of the breast in patients with postoperative scarring and silicon implants. J Comput Assist Tomogr 1990; 14:348–56.
5. Kaiser WA, Zeitler E. MR imaging of the breast: fast imaging sequences with and without Gd-DTPA. Radiology 1989; 170: 681–686.
6. Lewis-Jones HG, Whitehouse GH, Leinster SJ. The role of MRI in the assessment of local recurrent breast carcinoma. Clin Radiol 1991; 43:197–204.
7. Orel S, Schnall MD, LiVolsi VA, Troupin RH. Suspicious breast lesions: MR imaging with radiologic-pathologic correlation. Radiology 1994; 190:485–493.
8. Heywang-Kobrunner SH. Contrast-enhanced magnetic resonance imaging of the breast. Invest Radiol 1994; 29:94–104.
9. Sinha S, Sinha U, Lufkin R, Hanafee W. Technical note: pulse sequence optimization for use with a biopsy needle in MRI. Magn Reson Imaging 1989; 7:575–579.

10. Duckwiler G, Lufkin R, Teresi L, et al. Head and neck lesions: MR-guided aspiration biopsy. Radiology 1989; 170:519–522.

11. Lufkin R, Teresi L, Hanafee W. New needle for MR-guided aspiration cytology of the head and neck. Am J Roentgenol 1987; 149:380–382.

12. Lufkin R, Teresi L, Chiu L, Hanafee W. A technique for MR guided needle placement in the head and neck. Am J Roentgenol 1988; 151:193–196.

13. Lufkin R, Duckwiler G, Spickler E, et al. Technical note: MR body stereotaxis: an aid for MR guided biopsies. J Comput Assist Tomogr 1988; 12:1088–1089.

14. Lufkin R, Layfield L. Coaxial needle system for MR and CT guided aspiration cytology. J Comput Assist Tomogr 1989; 13:1105–1107.

15. Fischer U, Vosshenrich R, Keating D, et al. MR-guided biopsy of suspect breast lesions with a simple stereotaxic add-on device for surface coils. Radiology 1994; 192:272–273.

16. Schnall MD, Orel SG, Connick TJ. MR guided biopsy of the breast. MRI Clin North Am 1994; 2:585–589.

17. Sinha S, Gorczyca DP, DeBruhl ND, et al. MR imaging of silicone breast implants: Comparison of different coil arrays. Radiology 1993;187:284–286.

12

PATHOLOGIC
CONSIDERATIONS

Bruce J. Youngson
Paul Peter Rosen

Close communication among the radiologist, pathologist, surgeon, and oncologist has become essential in the multidisciplinary climate of current clinical practice. Interventional radiologic breast procedures now encompass fine needle aspiration biopsy (FNAB), core biopsy, and needle/wire localization procedures, which may be x-ray or ultrasound guided. This chapter considers each of these procedures from a pathologist's perspective.

FINE NEEDLE ASPIRATION BIOPSY OF BREAST LESIONS

FNAB of the breast has been practiced for more than 50 years and is often the first diagnostic procedure performed in the clinical investigation of a breast lesion. The breast is especially suited to this method of diagnosis because cytologic samples can be obtained rapidly and with minimal patient preparation. FNAB is a relatively simple procedure that can be performed in an office setting. Sample preparation is fast and technically uncomplicated, facilitating prompt diagnosis, which, if positive, makes it possible to discuss therapeutic options in the same patient visit. For patients with clinically advanced disease, the diagnosis of carcinoma by FNAB may avoid an open surgical biopsy.

In describing his experience with FNAB in the breast, Stewart concluded in 1933, "... It must not be inferred that diagnosis is always simple and that no errors have been made. Until the pathologist has familiarized himself with the various pitfalls, errors are certain to occur."[1] That statement is as true today as it was in 1933. Skill in performing FNAB and expertise in its interpretation depends on continued experience with substantial numbers of cases.

The diagnostic results of an FNAB must not be taken out of clinical context. Aspiration is generally regarded as one part of a triad of investigations, which also involves mammographic findings and physical examination of the breast. Treatment should not be recommended or undertaken on the basis of a positive FNAB unless supported by clinical studies. Some authors have concluded that FNAB is a cost-effective procedure for the management of palpable breast lesions because it can be relied on as a substitute for more costly surgical biopsy.[2,3] This point remains controversial, however, and other authors recommend that a positive FNAB diagnosis be confirmed by a tissue biopsy.[4,5] This confirmation is particularly important when dealing with nonpalpable lesions because treatment depends heavily on a detailed assessment of the histologic features of the lesion. Furthermore, few centers presently have substantial experience with interpreting the cytology of nonpalpable breast lesions, which often present a challenging diagnostic problem even in histologic sections. Occasionally, the integrity of small lesions may be altered as a result of the needle localization or aspiration biopsy procedure, particularly if there have been several passes.

A surgical biopsy should be performed despite a nondiagnostic cytology report whenever clinical or mammographic features of the lesion indicate a significant abnormality. Delay in diagnosis attributed to false-negative benign and acellular aspirates has been a particular problem in young women because of the relatively high frequency of benign disease and low sensitivity of mammography in this group. Although carcinoma cells are much more likely to be present in the aspirate from a tumor regarded clinically to be carcinoma, Bell et al.[6] reported that surgical biopsies revealed carcinoma in 36 percent of clinically "suspicious" aspirated lesions, in 20 percent regarded as clinically significant, and in 3 percent of specimens from lesions diagnosed clinically as benign. In another series, 8 percent of clinically benign lesions that yielded a cytologically negative aspirate proved to be carcinoma when biopsied surgically.[7]

False-positive diagnoses have been remarkably infrequent, ranging from 0 to 1.3 percent and rarely exceeding 0.3 percent.[8] In most institutions, the frequency of error does not differ from experience with frozen sections in general or with frozen sections of breast tumors in particular. Inexperience is a signifi-

cant contributing factor when a false-positive diagnosis is made. It is essential that a high threshold be maintained based on stringent diagnostic criteria to minimize such errors. Diagnostic material should be abundant and present on at least two separate slides. Although a criterion, cellularity is not by itself sufficient for a diagnosis because substantial amounts of benign epithelium may be obtained from papillomas, fibroadenomas, and other benign lesions. The epithelium from a benign lesion usually forms cohesive sheets or clusters, whereas cells from carcinomas tend to separate and appear dispersed (Fig. 12-1). Other features significantly associated with carcinoma are clustering with fewer than 15 cells per group, irregular nuclear contours, nucleoli, and cellular debris in the background.

A benign diagnosis is suggested by monolayers of more than 15 cells, nuclei with smooth contours smaller than twice the diameter of an erythrocyte, and absence of nucleoli. Aspirates from the lactating breast, gynecomastia, and various proliferative duct lesions (e.g., atypical papillomatosis) constitute significant diagnostic hazards. The aspirate from a granular cell tumor, which clinically simulates carcinoma, can be misinterpreted easily as carcinoma if the cytologist does not notice granules dispersed on the slide from disrupted cells. Technically imperfect prepara-

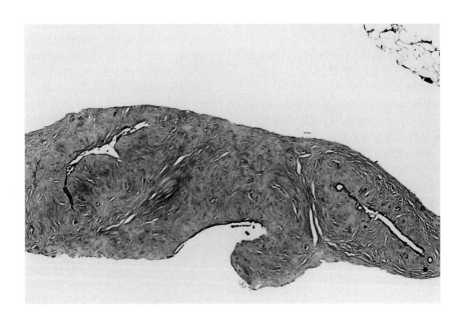

Fig. 12-1. Core biopsy. Sample of a fibroadenoma obtained after stereotaxic localization with a 14-gauge needle. Note epithelial lined clefts and dense stroma. (H & E × 40).

tions, particularly those with drying artifacts, should be interpreted with extreme caution.

Cystic Lesions

One of the most important and practical uses of FNAB is to distinguish a fluid-filled cyst from a solid tumor of the breast. In most instances, aspiration of cyst contents is therapeutic as well as diagnostic. During aspiration, the cyst collapses, and in most cases, much of the epithelial lining is stripped from the supporting stroma and removed in the aspirate. Because reaccumulation of fluid rarely occurs in such cases, it has been presumed that the epithelium contributed to the fluid formation and that in the absence of epithelium, the cystic space is effaced by the adherent, exposed, apposing stromal surfaces.

The need for routine cytologic examination of aspirated breast cyst fluid is controversial. The frequency of carcinoma among cystic lesions from which material was submitted for cytology examination in three studies was 2 percent in 1,714 specimens.[6,9,10] The majority of the carcinomas were associated with bloody fluid and/or a residual mass. As a consequence, it would appear that in the absence of the latter clinical findings, microscopic examination of cyst fluid is not mandatory. However, consideration should be given to other factors such as a past history of breast carcinoma, significant atypia on previous biopsy, or a family history of breast carcinoma, which may indicate that the patient is at increased risk for breast cancer.

Cytologic examination of cyst fluid is essential in some circumstances. A bloody or serosanguinous aspirate should be examined microscopically. Bright red blood may be indicative of a traumatic aspiration with hemorrhage into the cyst, resulting in a persistent mass. Regardless of the character of the fluid obtained, the presence of a residual mass immediately after aspiration requires cytologic examination of the specimen. Reaccumulation of fluid in a cyst, particularly within a short period of time, is an indication for cytologic study of the second aspirate. In some cases, regardless of the cytologic findings, excisional biopsy is necessary, especially for aspirates that yield bloody fluid or are associated with a mass.

The microscopic findings in breast cyst fluid vary considerably. Many specimens are nearly acellular, especially if no effort has been made to concentrate the material by centrifugation or filtration. In a cellular specimen, benign epithelial cells occur singly or in small groups, and histiocytes ("foam cells"), lymphocytes, and epithelial cells exhibiting apocrine features are found in varying proportions. Clustered cells generally indicate papillary proliferation of epithelium lining the cyst, an especially frequent finding when there is apocrine metaplasia. Standard cytologic criteria are applied to the diagnosis of cells obtained in a cyst aspirate.

Solid Lesions

FNAB of solid breast tumors is now an established diagnostic procedure. Numerous studies have been conducted to evaluate the accuracy and clinical utility of the aspiration cytology diagnosis of breast carcinoma. The primary role of this procedure is to provide a prompt diagnosis of a palpable breast tumor in young women, among whom the frequency of carcinoma is extremely low. The introduction of a reliable FNAB program in a hospital or clinic is likely to reduce the frequency of benign surgical biopsies. The decision not to perform a surgical biopsy on the basis of a negative FNAB, however, requires careful consideration of the clinical and mammographic findings.

The frequency with which carcinoma has been diagnosed in various series depends on the selection of patients, as well as the skill of the personnel who perform and interpret the FNAB. The sensitivity of FNAB (proportion of histologically proven carcinomas detected cytologically) has ranged from 69 to 96 percent in some of the larger published series.[6,9,10] False-negative reports (proportion of carcinomas not detected cytologically) are the result of scanty, improperly prepared, or poorly preserved samples of the lesion; aspirates of lesions that present inherent diagnostic problems (e.g., papillary carcinoma versus papilloma), and aspirates that have missed the lesion entirely. Attempts to aspirate palpable tumors smaller than 2 cm or those located deeply in large breasts, indistinct lesions, and nonpalpable abnormalities detected by mammography are more likely to result in false-negative diagnoses.

Daum et al.[11] reported a sensitivity of 57 percent when nonpalpable mammographically detected lesions were diagnosed by a "scouting needle" technique in the physician's office without radiologic localization. The yield in such cases has been improved by using mammographically or stereotaxically guided procedures to ensure placement of the aspiration needle in the lesion. The sensitivity of stereotaxic FNAB of nonpalpable lesions ranges from 78 to 100 percent, and the specificity is usually 100 percent.[12-15] False-negative specimens are often associated with lobular carcinoma in situ, intraductal carcinoma, or with lesions detected only on the basis of calcifications.[12,14] The sensitivity of the procedure for palpable mass lesions is close to 100 percent. Ultrasound also has been used to localize lesions for FNAB in various organs, including the breast.[16]

It is possible to identify some specific histologic types of breast carcinoma from an FNAB specimen. The aspirate from infiltrating lobular carcinoma may be relatively scanty, and it is generally composed of small isolated cells with sparse cytoplasm. Occasionally, the cells are arranged in the characteristic linear "single file" fashion, as seen in tissue sections. Tubular carcinoma may be suspected when the aspirate contains clusters of cells that are arranged in an angular glandular configuration, but these lesions are difficult to diagnose because of the absence of cytologic atypia. Aspirates from infiltrating lobular and tubular carcinomas are more likely to be nondiagnostic than are specimens from ordinary infiltrating duct carcinomas. Abundant extracellular mucin characterizes the aspirate from mucinous carcinoma, whereas a specimen from a medullary carcinoma typically has poorly differentiated tumor cells scattered among numerous lymphocytes and plasma cells. Papillary carcinoma typically features three-dimensional clusters of tumor cells, as well as dispersed single cells. Apocrine carcinoma cells are most easily recognized when there is prominent cytoplasmic eosinophilia, but some apocrine carcinomas exhibit striking cytoplasmic clearing. Metaplastic carcinoma may be suspected when the specimen is highly cellular and contains abundant pleomorphic cells. A variant of metaplastic carcinoma, mammary carcinoma with osteoclast-like giant cells, can be readily diagnosed in an FNAB specimen if the osteoclast-like cells containing multiple cytologically benign nuclei are identified. These cells are acid phosphatase positive, a property not shared by carcinomatous multinucleated giant cells in metaplastic carcinomas.

Distinguishing between some types of carcinoma and benign lesions may be difficult. This problem is most likely to be encountered with well-differentiated invasive duct carcinoma and cytologically low-grade forms of intraductal carcinoma. The FNAB specimens obtained from such lesions often have abundant cohesive clusters of uniform cells with cytologically bland nuclei. Honeycombing may occur in cohesive sheets of cells from cribriform carcinoma.

Benign lesions can mimic patterns associated with various tumor types. Fibroadenomas with myxoid degeneration may give rise to an FNAB specimen that can be mistaken for mucinous carcinoma. In most instances, a careful search for stromal cell elements and the cytologically bland appearance of the epithelial component displayed as flat sheets of cells in the FNAB from a fibroadenoma provide sufficient evidence for reliably distinguishing between mucinous carcinoma and a fibroadenoma. Cells in mucinous carcinoma are atypical and arranged in three-dimensional groups. It is essential, therefore, to establish the presence of carcinoma cells before attempting to classify the lesion. Cytologic atypia associated with pregnancy produces a confusing picture in an FNAB specimen that can result in a false-positive interpretation. The benign lesions most often encountered in pregnant women are a galactocele, lactational adenoma, and fibroadenoma with lactational change. The aspirate from a galactocele tends to be sparsely cellular with degenerating cells and foamy histiocytes, whereas a lactational adenoma gives rise to a highly cellular specimen.

In addition to routine cytologic examination, needle aspiration specimens also can be used to study tumor cells for hormone receptors[17,18] and other tumor markers. A close correlation has been found between the assessment of hormone receptors in FNAB[17,18] or drill biopsy specimens[21] and biochemical analysis of the tissues. FNAB specimens also have been used for serial studies of oncogene amplification during the course of chemotherapy.[20] Using procedures such as slot-blot hybridization and polymerase chain reaction, it may be possible to obtain useful information from relatively scanty specimens.

CORE BIOPSY OF BREAST LESIONS

During the last decade interest has grown in the use of core needle biopsies for the diagnosis of solid tumors as an alternative to FNAB. This diagnostic method has become especially attractive with the availability of cutting needles and automated biopsy guns. The specimen obtained by this method consists of slender cylindrical fragments or cores of tissue, which can be used to make frozen as well as paraffin sections. At Memorial Sloan-Kettering Cancer Center, the cores of tissue are placed immediately in 10 percent formalin, fixed, paraffin embedded, and stained with hematoxylin and eosin (H & E). Tissue preparation can be accomplished with one day "turnaround time." The presence or absence of microcalcifications is assessed by specimen radiography, which is correlated with the mammographic findings. One survey found that most pathologists questioned had more experience in examining tissue sections and, therefore, found interpretation of needle core biopsies to be easier than the evaluation of aspiration cytology specimens.[21] Core biopsy specimens allow the assessment of both histologic and cytologic features; therefore, unlike FNAB, they can differentiate invasive from in situ carcinoma (Fig. 12-2). In one study, larger samples obtained with a 14-gauge needle and automated gun proved more reliable for diagnosis than those obtained from 18-gauge needles.[22] Needle core biopsies also can provide reliable samples for hormone-receptor analysis.

The increasing use of stereotaxic-guided FNAB and core biopsy has made it possible to sample reliably a growing number of nonpalpable, radiographically detected lesions. In one series of 100 such lesions of at least 5 mm in diameter, large-core needle biopsy correctly identified 35 of 36 carcinomas confirmed on open surgical biopsy.[23] When the lesions under investigation contain microcalcifications, radiologic examination of the needle core specimen (specimen radiography) is a useful method for documenting that calcifications are included in the sample. Stereotaxic biopsy also makes it possible to obtain cytologic specimens for immunocytochemical hormone receptor analysis from mammographically detected nonpalpable lesions.

The reported range of true positive diagnoses of carcinoma obtained by core needle biopsy (67 to 89 percent) approaches that reported with the drill biopsy (75 to 99 percent) or aspiration cytology (69 to 96

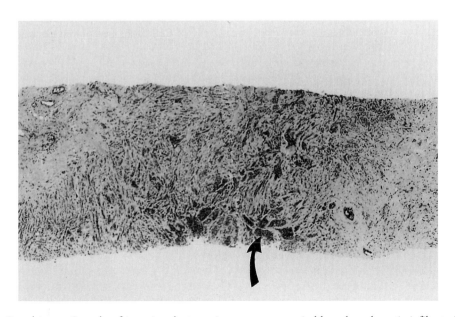

Fig. 12-2. Core biopsy. Sample of invasive duct carcinoma accompanied by a lymphocytic infiltrate in the midportion of the specimen. Some groups of carcinoma cells are marked with an *arrow*. (H & E × 40).

percent).[21,24-30] Studies that demonstrated a higher frequency of true positive diagnoses with needle biopsy than with aspiration cytology[24,31] have had remarkably poor results with the latter procedure (52 and 42 percent positive rates, respectively) and have studied very few patients (119 and 60 patients, respectively). In one study of 50 women with malignant breast tumors, the frequency of positive diagnosis by aspiration cytology was slightly higher than that obtained with needle biopsy (76 versus 69 percent).[32]

False-negative diagnoses by needle biopsy reflect problems in sampling and tissue preservation comparable to those encountered in aspiration biopsy. In addition to failure to enter the lesion, diagnostic material may not be obtained from carcinomas in which there is considerable necrosis or desmoplastic fibrosis. Neoplastic cells in some tumors are particularly susceptible to distortion by the biopsy procedure ("crush artifact") and may be uninterpretable. The yield is improved if more than one pass of the needle is made in the lesion, with the best results obtained in one series with three or four passes.[33] In general, false-negative results have been less common with FNAB than with needle biopsy.[8]

The potential for a false-positive core needle biopsy diagnosis exists, particularly with sclerosing adenosis and sclerosing ductal proliferations, such as the so-called "radial scar." Mingling of proliferating epithelium and stroma in these tumors often simulates the appearance of invasive carcinoma. Although this configuration, referred to as *pseudoinvasion*, generally can be appreciated in a tissue section of the entire lesion, the small sample obtained by needle core biopsy might be misinterpreted as carcinoma. The hazard is especially great when dealing with frozen section material in which the quality of cytologic detail is less than in paraffin sections. We believe that performing frozen sections on needle biopsy specimens of the breast is inappropriate because of the risk of diagnostic misinterpretations and problems in making satisfactory sections. Follow-up open biopsy is warranted in cases showing sclerosing lesions. As with FNAB, interpretation of core biopsies in the context of clinical and mammographic findings is essential to the appropriate management of these lesions. Core biopsies showing epithelial atypia and/or lobular carcinoma in situ, for example, may then be managed with close clinical follow-up or biopsy as the individual situation warrants.

NEEDLE/WIRE LOCALIZED BREAST SPECIMENS

Carcinoma is found in approximately 25 percent of nonpalpable breast lesions biopsied because of suspicious mammographic findings. To effectively evaluate a mammographically directed breast biopsy, it is necessary to have a specimen radiograph and the clinical mammogram available simultaneously. A variety of procedures have been described in the literature for specimen radiography; this chapter will not address their relative merit, which depends on the availability of personnel and other resources in a given institution. Regardless of whether the interpretation of specimen radiographs is the responsibility of a pathologist or a radiologist, however, certain general principles do apply.

The surgical biopsy should be performed using sharp dissection rather than with a cautery scalpel to avoid thermal artifacts that interfere with histologic assessment and hormone receptor analysis.

A radiograph should be made of the intact excisional biopsy specimen, and the film compared with the patient's mammogram before the specimen in sectioned. If the tissue is dissected before obtaining a specimen radiograph, the sectioning may disrupt the pattern of calcifications and interfere with comparison of the clinical and specimen films.

In the absence of an obvious gross lesion, it is unwise to select a random sample for frozen section before specimen radiography. If the biopsy was performed for calcifications and the specimen fails to show them, it will be necessary to radiograph the frozen section sample. It is also theoretically possible to lose calcifications in tissue trimmed away in the process of preparing the frozen tissue.

In one study of 359 mammographically detected lesions, frozen section yielded a correct diagnosis in 68 percent of cases; 17.3 percent did not have a frozen section, 1.9 percent of frozen sections yielded false-negative results, and 0.6 percent had false-positive diagnoses.[34] It is recommended that mammographically detected lesions be processed for paraffin sections and that frozen sections be performed only in exceptional situations.

The immediate goal of specimen radiography is to confirm that a nonpalpable lesion with calcifications has been excised. This procedure should be determined intraoperatively because if the lesion is not present in the specimen, the surgeon may elect to perform an additional biopsy. Missed lesions have been reported by specimen radiography in up to 13.6 percent of needle localization biopsies,[35] but in most series, lesions have been missed in 5 percent or less of cases.[36-38]

False-negative specimen radiographs may occur because the lesion has been distorted by the surgery, by dissection of the specimen after excision, or as a result of improper positioning of the specimen when the image was obtained. The specimen radiograph also may fail to contain the lesion because of inaccurate preoperative localization or migration of the localizing wire or needle in the breast before the biopsy is performed. Finally, if localization has not been performed, the surgeon may misjudge the position of the mass or calcifications on the basis of conventional mammographic views. Cutaneous calcifications can be misinterpreted as an intraparenchymal lesion.[39] Because skin is not normally removed during surgery, these calcifications will not be contained in the specimen. Tangential views and stereotaxic imaging are useful for localizing the cutaneous position of such calcifications. One unusual cutaneous abnormality that may mimic calcifications in the breast is a skin tattoo.[40] Tattoo powder applied to specimens inadvertently or purposefully to mark margins is sometimes a source of factitious microcalcifications that may interfere with the interpretation of specimen radiographs.[41]

The procedure utilized to localize a lesion preoperatively may affect the ability of the pathologist to analyze the specimen. If a dye injection with methylene blue is used, some laboratory evidence suggests that it may significantly lower estrogen receptor levels[42]; this problem does not occur when the dye toluidine (isosulfan) blue is used.[43] These conclusions have been based on in vitro studies in which the dyes were added to the cytosols in the laboratory. One clinical study, however, reported that 62.5 percent of carcinomas localized by the methylene blue dye method did not differ notably from the frequency of receptor positivity among carcinomas excised without localization.[44]

Localization procedures also may assist the pathologist in locating the lesion for pathologic study. Before the position of the specimen is changed, the site of the calcifications should be identified grossly.

This portion of the tissue should be excised from the specimen and labeled. The remainder of the tissue also should be dissected, because occasionally the calcifications have proved to be in a benign process near an unanticipated carcinoma fortuitously included in the excisional biopsy.

Calcifications in mammographically directed breast biopsies should be sought in histologic sections of the tissue, and the microscopic report should specify the pathologic changes associated with these calcifications. Microcalcifications found in breast tissue have been thoroughly described and classified by Frappart et al.[45,46] The majority of calcifications detected in mammograms are basophilic concretions of varying size composed of calcium phosphates, largely in the form of hydroxyapatite. These type II calcifications of Frappart are not birefringent. The less frequent type I calcifications composed of calcium oxalate dihydrate crystals (Weddellite) are birefringent, nonbasophilic, von Kossa-negative crystals. These colorless calcium oxalate crystals are difficult to identity on H & E stained sections with regular light microscopy. They tend to fragment and may be mixed with secretory debris, sometimes accompanied by multinucleated giant cells. Such fragmented crystals are easily mistaken for holes in the section, but they usually have angular rather than round contours.

In one series, 13.6 percent (9/66) of mammographically detected calcifications identified histologically consisted of calcium oxalate crystals (type I), 72.7 percent (48/66) were calcium phosphate (type II), and 13.6 percent were a mixture of types I and II.[47] Similar frequencies have been found by other investigators.[48] A reliable method for distinguishing between type I and type II calcifications in vivo is not available on mammography.

Once it has been established that the mammographically detected lesion is present in the biopsy specimen radiograph, the surgical margins of the specimen should be marked with ink, dye, silver nitrate, or whatever is used in a particular institution to indicate a margin. The specimen may then be sectioned at approximately 3-mm intervals, the slices numbered and resubmitted for mammography. The mammographically suspicious areas are indicated and embedded in toto for microscopic examination along with representative samples of the remaining tissue.

EPITHELIAL DISPLACEMENT IN SURGICAL BREAST SPECIMENS AFTER NEEDLING PROCEDURES

Aspiration biopsy was introduced initially as an alternative to incisional surgical biopsy because of concern that trauma associated with the latter procedure could result in vascular dissemination of tumor cells.[49] The presence of circulating tumor cells has been documented repeatedly in patients with a variety of cancers including mammary carcinoma.[50-53] This phenomenon has been observed when there has been no manipulation of tumor, but evidence suggests that more cells may be dispersed after palpation or biopsy.[52] The prognostic significance of circulating tumor cells is uncertain. Some investigators have reported no demonstrable effect on survival.[52] Whether breast needling procedures contribute more or less than surgical biopsy to the hematogenous or lymphatic dispersal of tumor cells has not been specifically determined. Two studies of patients who presented with palpable invasive carcinoma, however, failed to find any difference in the survival between breast cancer patients whose diagnosis was based on FNAB and those who underwent surgical biopsy. [54,55]

More recently, concern has again been expressed about the potential for complications and diagnostic problems that may be attributed to FNAB or needle core biopsies of the breast. Although another advantage often cited for FNAB and core biopsy is the lack of the postsurgical changes that complicate the interpretation of follow-up mammograms, alterations in benign breast lesions caused by FNAB have been reported to result in ultrasound findings that mimic carcinoma.[56] Consequently, ultrasound examinations should be performed before an invasive procedure such as FNAB.

A variety of needling procedures including fine needle aspiration, core biopsy, needle/wire localization, suture placement, and/or infiltration with local anesthetic may lead to dislodgement and displacement of fragments of breast epithelium into tissue away from the target lesion of the needling procedure. Displaced fragments of benign and malignant ductal epithelium have been observed lying in breast stroma and within vascular channels in breast specimens obtained subsequent to the needling proce-

dure.[57-61] These displaced epithelial fragments mimic stromal invasion to a variable degree and represent a potential source of misdiagnosis. The biologic significance of epithelial displacement in this setting is unknown.

Evidence of a recent needling procedure in breast tissue is most often suggested by areas of tissue disruption with hemorrhage, inflammation, fat necrosis, and/or a granulation tissue-like reaction in the breast stroma. A microscopically identifiable needle track may be present. Sloughed and disrupted epithelium, sometimes accompanied by intraductal and intralobular hemorrhage, has been observed frequently in close proximity to the area of needle-track hemorrhage. Among the cases we have seen, the most common phenomenon is the presence of displaced epithelial fragments in fibrous breast stroma or fat, adjacent to, or within the needle track (Fig. 12-3). Histologic findings suggesting epithelial displacement include the presence of scattered, isolated fragments of breast epithelium in artificial spaces within breast stroma, accompanied by hemorrhage, fat necrosis, inflammation, hemosiderin-laden macrophages, or granulation tissue. Morphologically, these displaced fragments of epithelium mimic stromal invasion to a variable degree, but they tend not to have the intimate association with stroma that true invasive carcinoma demonstrates as it grows within breast stroma.

Few studies have investigated the incidence of the phenomenon of epithelial displacement following needling. Boppana et al.[60] reviewed 100 consecutive breast carcinomas that had been subjected to prior FNAB and noted displaced epithelial fragments in 36 percent of cases.[60] Youngson et al.[61] reviewed slides from 43 consecutive cases in which surgical biopsy and/or mastectomy had been performed after an initial stereotaxic 14-gauge core biopsy diagnosis of breast carcinoma and identified displaced epithelial fragments outside of the main tumor mass in 12 of 43 (28 percent) cases.[61] However, multiple needling procedures (e.g., local anesthetic injection in all 43 cases, needle localization in 22 of 43 cases, suture placement in 18 of 43 cases, and FNAB in 1 of 43 cases) had been performed in each of the cases reviewed.

Few authors have commented on the morphologic changes in breast tissue described earlier. In a series of more than 10,000 breast lesions subjected to FNAB (23-gauge needle), Us-Krasovec et al.[62] reported that

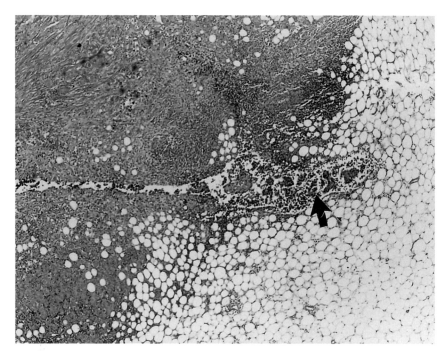

Fig. 12-3. Needle track in biopsy. Infiltrating duct carcinoma (left) invading fat (right). Needle track is the horizontal defect in the tissue from the left border. *Arrow* indicates fragments of carcinoma displaced into needle track. (H & E × 100).

tissue injury was infrequent, consisting only of small areas of hemorrhage. Other studies of FNAB-associated changes in the breast have been limited largely to case reports. Tabbara et al.[57] described a single post-FNAB specimen with extensive intraductal carcinoma, in which clusters of intact, abnormal epithelial cells were present in an inflammatory background in the needle track, simulating stromal invasion. Harter et al.[58] also reported a single case in which fragments of mucinous carcinoma were identified in the needle track of a wire localized breast biopsy specimen that had been subjected to stereotaxic 14-gauge core needle biopsy 2 weeks earlier. Grabau et al.[59] found carcinoma cells along a needle track in the skin of a mastectomy specimen after invasive carcinoma had been diagnosed by core needle biopsy 26 days earlier. In a follow-up study, these authors[59] reviewed 47 mastectomy specimens in which breast carcinoma had been previously diagnosed by 19-gauge Surecut (TSK Modified Menghini Aspiration Biopsy Set) core needle biopsy. They looked specifically at the needle track in the skin and adjacent subcutis rather than searching for displaced epithelium in the breast tissue itself and found carcinoma cells along the needle track in two cases (4 percent). On the basis of this observation, they recommended that surgeons excise the needle track and avoid penetration of thoracic wall muscle during breast needling procedures because of the potential for seeding tumor cells into these tissues.

The issue of tumor cell dissemination after needle biopsy also has been examined in several different target organs, including the breast. Although a theoretical risk exists, the actual documented risk appears to be small, correlating with the gauge of needle used.[63,64] How displaced fragments of epithelium behave biologically and whether they have the potential to remain viable and grow after dissemination are unanswered questions.

Few studies have investigated the possible clinical relevance of the preceding findings. Berg and Robbins[54] looked at patients with stage-matched palpable invasive breast cancers treated by mastectomy after diagnosis by aspiration biopsy or open biopsy, respectively, and found no difference in 15-year survival rates.[54] Kopans et al.[65] reviewed 74 women with nonpalpable breast cancer who had surgery after needle localization and found no evidence of subsequent local recurrence that could be attributed to the needle localization procedure. Fajardo[66] criticized this study, pointing out that a majority of the patients were not treated with breast-conserving surgery and thus were not prone to needle track recurrence because the needle track had likely been resected with the mastectomy specimen. The same criticism applies to the study by Berg and Robbins.[54]

We have seen the phenomenon of tumor cell displacement in the setting of a number of different needling procedures including wire/needle localization, FNAB, core biopsy, suture placement, and local anesthetic injection, and over a wide range of types and gauges (14 to 25 gauge) of needles and wires. The physical disruption of tissue resulting from the trauma of introducing a needle or wire through breast tissue, with or without the additional barotrauma of applied suction or injection of local anesthetic, may explain the phenomenon of epithelial displacement into stroma. With tissue disruption, lymphatic or vascular channels also may be breached, allowing detached epithelial cells to enter vascular channels and perhaps even to be transported to lymph nodes draining this area.[61] Whether these displaced fragments remain viable, representing, in the case of malignant epithelium, potential metastatic deposits, is not known.

In patients undergoing mastectomy after large-core needle biopsy, the needle track is usually resected with the breast; thus, concerns about local recurrence due to needle track seeding are probably not warranted for patients treated by this procedure. Although dissemination of tumor cells into lymphatics at the time of core biopsy may occur, the clinical significance of this phenomenon is unknown and may be largely theoretical. Animal experiments with solid tumors suggest that only 1 in 10,000 (0.01 percent) circulating tumor cells eventually are able to settle out and grow as metastatic tumor deposits.[67,68]

The phenomenon of epithelial displacement in surgical breast specimens that follows needling procedures may be encountered with increasing frequency in general surgical pathology practice as the trend toward needle-based diagnosis increases. These alterations present the pathologist with a challenging diagnostic problem. A malignant diagnosis should not be based solely on the appearance of epithelium within stroma because epithelial displacement has been observed after needling procedures in several benign breast lesions, notably papillary duct hyperplasia and intraductal papilloma. The significance of carcinomatous lymphovascular emboli is uncertain in the setting described previously. Until further information becomes available, we have interpreted the finding of lymphatic tumor emboli as evidence of invasion in patients with in situ carcinoma, even when conventional stromal invasion cannot be identified. We also have regarded clusters of carcinoma cells in the lymph node capsule or subcapsular sinus associated with such emboli as metastatic carcinoma. Such foci may be mistakenly diagnosed as benign ectopic mammary glands.

Eliciting a history of previous needling procedure may help prevent histopathologic confusion and an erroneous tissue diagnosis in cases such as those described here. Further studies are necessary to clarify the biologic significance of these phenomena.

REFERENCES

1. Stewart FW. The diagnosis of tumors by aspiration. Am J Pathol 1933; 9:801–811.
2. Layfield LJ, Chrischilles EA, Cohen MB, Bottles K. The palpable breast nodule. A cost-effectiveness analysis of alternate diagnostic approaches. Cancer 1993; 72:1642–1651.
3. Koss LG. The palpable breast nodule: a cost-effectiveness analysis of alternate diagnostic approaches. The role of the needle aspiration biopsy. Cancer 1993; 72:1499–1502.
4. Lannin DR, Silverman JF, Pories WJ, Walker C. Cost-effectiveness of fine needle biopsy of the breast. Ann Surg 1986; 203:474–480.
5. Grant CS, Goellner JR, Welch JS, Martin JK. Fine-needle aspiration of the breast. Mayo Clin Proc 1986; 61:377–381.
6. Bell DA, Hajdu SI, Urban JA, Gaston JP. Role of aspiration cytology in the diagnosis and management of mammary lesions in office practice. Cancer 1983; 51:1182–1189.
7. Painter RW, Clark II WE, Deckers PJ. Negative findings on fine-needle aspiration biopsy of solid breast masses: patient management. Am J Surg 1988; 155:387–390.
8. Cusick JD, Dotan J, Jaecks RD, Boyle Jr WT. The role of Tru-cut needle biopsy in the diagnosis of carcinoma of the breast. Surg Gynecol Obstet 1990; 170:407–410.

9. Kline TS, Joshi LP, Neal HS. Fine needle aspiration of the breast. Diagnosis and pitfalls. A review of 3545 cases. Cancer 1979; 44:1458–1464.

10. Strawbridge HTG, Bassett AA, Foldes I. Role of cytology in management of lesions of the breast. Surg Gynecol Obstet 1981; 152:1–7.

11. Daum GS, Kline TS, Artymyshyn RL, Neal HS. Aspiration biopsy cytology of occult breast lesions by use of the "scouting needle." A prospective study of 261 cases. Cancer 1991; 67:2150–2152.

12. Layfield LJ, Parkinson B, Wong J, et al. Mammographically guided fine-needle aspiration biopsy of non-palpable breast lesions. Can it replace open biopsy? Cancer 1991; 68:2007–2011.

13. Teixidor HS, Wojtasek DA, Reiches EM, et al. Fine-needle aspiration of breast biopsy specimens: correlation of histologic and cytologic findings. Radiology 1992; 184:55–58.

14. Howell LP, Lindfors KK, Russell LA. Cytologic interpretation of fine-needle aspiration biopsies from clinically occult breast masses. Diagn Cytopathol 1991; 7:235–238.

15. Masood S, Frykberg ER, McLellan GL, et al. Prospective evaluation of radiologically directed fine-needle aspiration biopsy of nonpalpable breast lesions. Cancer 1990; 66:1480–1487.

16. Patel JJ, Gartell PC, Guyer PB, et al. Use of ultrasound localization to improve results of fine needle aspiration cytology of breast masses. J R Soc Med 1988; 81:10–12.

17. McClelland RA, Berger V, Wilson P, et al. Presurgical determination of estrogen receptor status using immunocytochemically stained fine needle aspirate smears in patients with breast cancer. Cancer Res 1987; 47:6118–6122.

18. Reiner A, Spona J, Reiner G, et al. Estrogen receptor analysis on biopsies and fine-needle aspirates from human breast carcinoma. Correlation of biochemical and immunohistochemical methods using antireceptor antibodies. Am J Pathol 1986; 125:443–449.

19. Noguchi S, Miyauchi K, Inaji H, et al. Enzyme immunoassay of estrogen and progesterone receptors in drill biopsy specimens from breast cancer. Eur J Clin Oncol 1989; 25:809–814.

20. Lonn U, Loun S, Nylen U, et al. Amplification of oncogenes in mammary carcinoma shown by fine-needle biopsy. Cancer 1991; 67:1396–1400.

21. Smeets HJ, Saltzstein SL, Meurer WT, Pilch YH. Needle biopsies in breast cancer diagnosis: techniques in search of an audience. J Surg Oncol 1986; 32:11–15.

22. McMahon AJ, Lutfy AM, Matthew A, et al. Needle core biopsy of the breast with spring-loaded device. Br J Surg 1992; 79:1042–1045.

23. Elvecrog EL, Lechner MC, Nelson MT. Nonpalpable breast lesions: correlation of stereotaxic large-core needle biopsy and surgical biopsy results. Radiology 1993; 188:453–455.

24. Elston CW, Cotton RE, Davies CJ, Blamey RW. A comparison of the use of the "Tru-Cut" needle and fine needle aspiration cytology in the pre-operative diagnosis of carcinoma of the breast. Histopathology 1978; 2:239–254.

25. Shabot MM, Goldberg IM, Schick P, et al. Aspiration cytology is superior to "Tru-Cut" needle biopsy in establishing the diagnosis of clinically suspicious breast masses. Ann Surg 1982; 196:122–126.

26. Roberts JG, Preece PE, Bolton PM, et al. The "tru-cut" biopsy in breast cancer. Clin Oncol 1975; 1:297–303.

27. Millis RR. Needle biopsy of the breast. In McDivitt RW, Oberman HA, Ozzello L, Kaufman N (eds). The Breast, Williams & Wilkins, Baltimore, 1984; 186–303.

28. Meyerowitz BR. Drill biopsy confirmation of breast cancer. Arch Surg 1976; 111:826–827.

29. McCormick JSTC, Shivas AA. Drill biopsy of the breast—a critical analysis. Br J Surg 1973; 60:953–956.

30. Minkowitz S, Moskowitz R, Khafif RA, Alderete MN. TRU-CUT needle biopsy of the breast. An analysis of its specificity and sensitivity. Cancer 1986; 57:320–323.

30. Sieinski W, Dabska M. Usefulness of drill biopsy in the diagnosis of breast tumors. Cancer 1976; 38:2567–2569.

31. Owen AWMC, Kumer EN. Migration of localizing wires used in guided biopsy of the breast. Clin Radiol 1991; 43:251.

32. Shabb N, Sneige N, Dekmezian RH. Myospherulosis. Fine needle aspiration cytologic findings in 19 cases. Acta Cytol 1991; 35:225–228.

33. Pennes DR, Naylor B, Rebner M. Fine needle aspiration biopsy of the breast. Influence of the number of passes and sample size on the diagnostic yield. Acta Cytol 1990; 34:673–676.

35. Norton LW, Zeligman BF, Pearlman NW. Accuracy and cost of needle localization breast biopsy. Arch Surg 1988; 123:945–950.

34. Tinnemans JGM, Wobbes T, Holland R, et al. Mammographic and histopathologic correlation of nonpalpable lesions of the breast and the reliability of frozen section diagnosis. Surg Gynecol Obstet 1987; 165:523–529.

36. Meyer JE, Sonnenfeld MR, Greene RA, Stomper PC. Preoperative localization of clinically occult breast lesions. Experience at a referral hospital. Radiology 1988; 169:627–628.

37. Symmonds Jr RF, Roberts JW. Management of nonpalpable breast abnormalities. Ann Surg 1987; 205:520–528.

38. Leis HP, Cammarata A, LaRaja RD, Higgins H. Breast biopsy and guidance for occult lesions. Int Surg 1985; 70:115–118.

39. Kopans DB, Meyer JE, Homer MJ, Grabbe J. Dermal deposits mistaken for breast calcifications. Radiology 1983; 149:592–594.

40. Brown RC, Zuehlke RL, Ehrhardt JC, Jochimsen PR. Tattoos simulating calcifications on xeroradiography of the breast. Radiology 1981; 138:583–584.

41. Lager DJ, O'Connor JC, Robinson RA, et al. Factitious microcalcifications in breast biopsy material: laboratory-induced error by use of tattoo powder for specimen mammography. J Surg Oncol 1989; 40:281–282.

42. Hirsch JI, Banks Jr WL, Sullivan JS, Horsley III JS. Effect of methylene blue on estrogen-receptor activity. Radiology 1989; 171:105–107.

43. Hirsch JI, Banks Jr WL, Sullivan JS, Horsley III JS. Noninterference of isosulfan blue on estrogen-receptor activity. Radiology 1989; 171:109–110.

44. Edeiken S, Suer WD, Vitale SF, et al. Needle localization of nonpalpable breast lesions using methylene blue. Breast Dis 1990; 3:75–80.

45. Frappart L, Boudeulle M, Boumendil J, et al. Structure and composition of microcalcifications in benign and malignant lesions of the breast. Hum Pathol 1984; 15:880–889.

46. Frappart L, Remy I, Hu CL, et al. Different types of microcalcifications observed in breast pathology. Correlations with histopathologic diagnosis and radiologic examination of operative specimens. Virchows Arch A 1986; 410:179–187.

47. Radi MJ. Calcium oxalate crystals in breast biopsies. An overlooked form of microcalcification associated with benign breast disease. Arch Pathol Lab Med 1989; 113:1367–1369.

48. Winston JS, Yeh I-T, Evers K, Friedman AK. Calcium oxalate is associated with benign breast tissue. Am J Clin Pathol 1993; 100:488–492.

49. Christopherson WM. Cytologic detection and diagnosis of cancer. Its contributions and limitations. Cancer 1983; 51:1201–1208.

50. Engell HC. Cancer cells in the circulating blood. A clinical study on the occurrence of cancer cells. Acta Chir Scand (Suppl) 1955; 201:1–70.

51. Romsdahl MM, Valaitis J, McGrath RG, McGrew EA. Circulating tumor cells in patients with carcinoma. JAMA 1965; 193:1087–1090.

52. Roger V, Brennhovd I, Hoeg K. Tumor cells in blood: the prognostic significance of tumor cells in blood during palpation and biopsy. Acta Cytol 1972; 16:557–560.

53. Shibata HR, Ritchie AC, Hopkirk JF, Long RC. Tumor cells in the circulating blood of patients with carcinoma of the breast and gastrointestinal tract. Can Med Assoc J 1963; 89:863–866.

54. Berg JW, Robbins GF. A late look at the safety of aspiration biopsy. Cancer 1962; 15:826–827.

55. Robbins GF, Brothers III JH, Eberhart WF, Quan S. Is aspiration biopsy of breast cancer dangerous to the patient? Cancer 1954; 7:774–788.

56. Svensson WE, Tohno E, Cosgrove DO, et al. Effects of fine-needle aspiration on the US appearance of the breast. Radiology 1992; 185:709–711.

57. Tabbara SO, Frierson HF, Fechner RE. Diagnostic problems in tissues previously sampled by fine-needle aspiration. Am J Clin Pathol 1991; 96:76–80.

58. Harter LP, Swengros Curtis J, Ponto G, Craig PH. Malignant seeding of the needle track during stereotaxic core needle biopsy. Radiology 1992; 185:713–714.

59. Grabau DA, Anderson JA, Gaverson HP, Dyneberg U. Needle biopsy of breast cancer. Appearance of tumor cells along the needle track. Eur J Surg Oncol 1993; 19:826–827.

60. Boppana S, May M, Hoda S. Does prior fine-needle-aspiration cause diagnostic difficulties in histologic evaluation of breast carcinomas? Lab Invest 1994; 70:13A.

61. Youngson BJ, Cranor M, Rosen PP. Epithelial displacement in surgical breast specimens following needling procedures. Am J Surg Pathol 1994; 18:896–903.

62. Us-Krasovec M, Golouh R, Auesperg M, Pogacnik A. Tissue damage after fine needle aspiration biopsy. Acta Cytol 1992; 36:456–457.

63. Roussel F, Dalion J. The risk of tumoral seeding in needle biopsies. Acta Cytol 1989; 33:936–938.

64. Smith EH. Complications of percutaneous abdominal fine-needle biopsy. Radiology 1991; 178:253–258.

65. Kopans DB, Gallagher WJ, Swann CA, et al. Does preoperative needle localization lead to an increase in local breast cancer recurrence? Radiology 1988; 167:667–668.

66. Fajardo LL. Breast tumor seeding along localization guide wire tracks. Radiology 1988; 169:580–581.

67. Liotta LA, Kleinerman J, Saidel GM. Quantitative relationships of intravascular tumor cells, tumor vessels, and pulmonary metastases following tumor implantation. Cancer Res 1974; 34:997–1003.

68. Schirrmacher B. Experimental approaches, theoretical concepts, and impacts for treatment strategies. Adv Cancer Res 1985; 43:1–32.

13

MEDICOLEGAL ASPECTS OF INTERVENTIONAL BREAST PROCEDURES

R. James Brenner

With the emergence of legislation in more than two thirds of the United States, as well as federal law endorsing reimbursement for screening mammography, a national commitment has been made for the early detection of breast cancer. Based in part on the results of clinical trials here and in Europe beginning in the late 1960s, such efforts are predicated on the contention that population-based screening and early detection will significantly decrease mortality rates from a disease that has been estimated to affect one in nine women during their lifetime.

Such optimism is tempered by several important developments. The first is a rise in the number of medical malpractice lawsuits instituted for the delay in diagnosis of breast cancer. In a 1995 study, the Physicians Insurer's Association of America (PIAA), a consortium of physician-owned insurance carriers, determined from lawsuit settlement data that such delay was the most common reason that physicians in general are sued and was the second leading source of indemnity payments.[1] The reasons for this statistic are multifactorial and have been reviewed elsewhere; in part, they are a result of the high expectations for early detection and cure by women in this country afflicted by breast cancer. These expectations are the result of information available from clinical studies.[2]

The second reason for caution is that the overall financial burden to society of diagnosing early breast cancer is necessarily increased by the cost of removing indeterminant breast lesions, the clinical or mammographic features of which are insufficiently specific when detected to exclude malignancy. In a study of 10 breast imaging centers participating in a regional low-cost screening mammography project in 1987, recommendations for further study or biopsy ranged from 5 to 33 percent; the higher limit was associated with the center that performed the most examinations.[2a]

Cost constraints imposed by emerging forms of reimbursement under managed care insurance plans have encouraged alternative approaches to customary excisional biopsy for suspicious lesions, in part because of the escalating depletion of resources associated with the larger number of biopsies generated from screening-detected breast abnormalities. The development of technology that allows more accurate evaluation and image-directed tissue sampling of breast lesions, as discussed elsewhere in this text, has been a timely response to such economic forces. Radiologists involved in interventional procedures enjoy an unprecedented opportunity to participate in patient care and management decisions that require the integration of clinical imaging and tissue sample information.

Enthusiasm for new breast interventional techniques is tempered by the medicolegal milieu in which medical malpractice lawsuits against radiologists in general are increasing significantly. For example, such lawsuits doubled in Texas between 1988 and 1992, and litigation may be escalating at an even faster rate against interventional radiologists.[3] A study from Boston observed that the cases filed against radiologic-related procedures accounted for a significant portion of indemnity payments.[4]

Unfortunately, the combination of high legal exposure for both breast cancer evaluation and interventional procedures in general has a negative impact on the efforts to combat breast cancer in a cost-effective manner. An understanding of basic legal principles and their application to the evolving role of the breast interventional radiologist should help in the formation of risk management and loss prevention strategies that permit responsible medical conduct and avoidance of a large number of malpractice lawsuits.

BASIC LEGAL PRINCIPLES

American law represents a combination of different legal fields or specialties, each with different rules of evidence and procedure. Criminal law, for example, represents the interests of society so that such cases are often denoted as "*State v ...*" or "*People v ....*" Because conviction may mean loss of civil liberties, the highest standards of proof are required. Physicians are rarely subject to such charges in standard medical practice, except in such extreme situations as misrepresentation to governmental agencies (e.g., Medicare fraud, or withdrawal of life support systems). Interestingly, attempts have been made in New York State to criminalize medical malpractice.[5]

Most medical malpractice cases come under the category of civil law and, more specifically, tort law. Tort law defines the relationships between or among individuals (or parties) where restitution is commonly sought, assessed as payment of money.

Civil law is derived from two sources: statutory law and common law. Statutory law is that body of law passed by lawmakers at the local, state, and national level, presumably representing a consensus of opinion by society of approved methods of conduct. Radiation safety provisions may be prescribed by local ordinances. Licensure laws and laws regarding different kinds of informed consent are usually governed by state law or jurisdictions. The Mammography Quality Standards Act (MQSA) was passed by Congress in 1992 and implemented in October 1994 as a national statutory law.[6] Most statutory law is

interpreted and implemented by regulatory agencies and under certain circumstances may be appealed for resolution to a court of law. For example, the Food and Drug Administration (FDA) is responsible for implementing MQSA, and its consideration of extending its jurisdiction to other aspects of breast imaging practices (e.g., stereotaxis) is a matter of interpretation because the statute does not expressly mention this technology.

Most law regarding medical malpractice is not covered by statutes and is referred to as common law. American common law, derived during the 18th century from English common law, embodies a series of decisions by judges and juries that is meant to establish proper parameters for conduct by individuals. Common law is based on a legal principle of *stare decisis*, whereby a decision rendered by an appellate court establishes legal precedent to be followed in that jurisdiction or locale when similar facts or situations arise. Appellate decisions and statutes are published for purposes of reference and, although binding only in the specific jurisdiction, may be relevant to other locales. The torts that are of importance to the breast interventional radiologist are battery and negligence, the latter associated with sometimes subtle implications. Each of these legal aspects of practice are examined from both an educational and risk-management perspective.

INTENTIONAL TORTS: BATTERY

Intentional torts may be defined as prohibited acts that one party intends to commit on another and that actually occur. Neither motive nor actual harm need be shown.

Battery is the unlawful nonconsensual and deliberate touching of another person and is thus an intentional tort. Incidental or normal touchings, such as in a crowded room, lack a sufficient intent to provide legal remedies. In fact, battery may be subject to both civil and criminal remedies, as in the case of a shooting, and illustrates perhaps the basis for seeking criminal penalties in certain medical procedures. In general, however, medical battery is tried under civil law.

Unpermitted touchings do not necessarily require expert opinion to establish their occurrence and thus lay judges or juries are often asked to make such determinations. Furthermore, intentional torts often are afforded punitive damages as a deterrent to such behavior. Most medical malpractice (professional liability) insurance policies do not provide indemnity for punitive damages.

INTENTIONAL TORTS: INFORMED CONSENT

A published survey of interventional breast procedures performed by radiologists largely consisting of preoperative needle localizations, cysts aspirations, and ductography found that a majority of radiologists do not obtain consent before performing these procedures.[7] The failure of radiologists to be sued for battery, except in rare instances, following these procedures may reflect the failure to win significant damages in these cases. This, in turn, causes a reticence of plaintiff attorneys—whose contingency fee is often predicated on a percent of collected monies to pursue such cases—to undertake such cases. The legal exposure of the radiologist under such circumstances nonetheless remains. For example, if the excisional removal of a image-localized breast lesion is unsuccessful—and a finite percentage of lesions fall into this category—the radiologist may then be sued together with the surgeon not only for negligence, but also for the battery involved in placing a needle into the breast without consent.

Liability in this setting is eliminated by obtaining consent to perform the procedure, which is based on the legal doctrine of *volenti non fit injuria* or "to he/she who consents there is not injury," which is a fundamental concept in the defense to a charge of battery. Any invasive procedure is a legal battery and, as mentioned, does not require a poor outcome for legal redress. The obtaining of proper consent defeats the legal complaint of battery.

It may be difficult to identify where "lawful touchings" in medicine end and battery begins. Many procedures, such as physical examination or simple phlebotomy, seem so inherent a part of clinical practice that courts recognize a form of implied consent when these procedures are performed, although even these issues have been the subject of controversy. In the practice of radiology, the assumption of consent for some procedures and the acknowledged need for consent for others are illustrated by the frequent recommendation to obtain informed consent for the administration of radiographic contrast material, but not for the venipuncture required to administer the material.[8]

A discussion of the law of consent and the many special types of consent applicable to a variety of medical situations is beyond the scope of this discussion and has been reviewed in depth elsewhere.[9] It is obvious, however, that the performance of interventional procedures requires informed consent, and the physician performing these procedures must understand the ramifications of this requirement. It is important to appreciate that exceeding the procedure for which consent has been given is considered a battery.

With the emergence of widespread screening mammography, an increasing number of mammographically detected lesions may be subject to interventional procedures. The frequency, complexity, and impact on patient management of such procedures require that physicians obtain appropriate informed consent before they begin invasive procedures. For example, if informed consent is obtained for aspiration of a questionable complex cyst and fluid cannot be evacuated, the radiologist is ill-advised to proceed with a subsequent large-bore core needle biopsy that may involve additional complications. Consent must be obtained for this new procedure. Because claims of duress may invalidate a consent, however, obtaining subsequent consent for a more invasive procedure while the patient is still undergoing an attempt at cyst aspiration may not be sufficient. Instead, if the possibility of additional intervention is anticipated, the initial consent should be sought for both procedures as a matter of contingency planning. Even this approach will be subject to scrutiny, as courts may look unfavorably on a situation where too many contingent procedures are sought by means of a single consent.

THE LAW OF NEGLIGENCE: GENERAL PRINCIPLES

The law of negligence governs most medical malpractice cases and is concerned with the conduct of physicians rather than the outcome of their actions. Nonetheless, it is the outcome, especially a negative outcome, that brings the issue of conduct to the court's attention. Unlike battery, intent is not a component of an analysis in negligence.

Common law notions of negligence emerged from decisions of judges that were directed toward those professions deemed to be providing a public calling, and these decisions are meant to provide for the safety and welfare of citizens. While the term *negligence* may be associated with a disparaging connotation, in law, it is a term of art, indicating a departure from accepted standards of care of the reasonable physician. Proof of negligence frequently requires expert testimony to establish the parameters of such standards of care. A case against a physician for negligence requires a showing of four elements: duty, breach of duty, causation, and damages.

Duty has been defined in the legal literature as: "One who undertakes gratuitously or for consideration to render services to another which he should recognize as necessary for the protection of the other person or things, is subject to liability to the other for physical harm resulting from his failure to exercise such care or perform is undertaking if such failure to exercise such care increased the risk of such harm..."[10] The measure by which care is evaluated is considered an objective standard: what a reasonable physician would do under similar circumstances. This standard may be considered in the context of a formula developed by one of the noted commentators in American jurisprudence, Judge Learned Hand, and is especially relevant to obtaining informed consent. Judge Hand suggested that the standard of care be measured as the product of the severity of an untoward event and its likelihood.

The second element of negligence is breech of duty, or breech of the standard of care.

The third element is causation. If the defendant's actions are the "cause in fact" and "proximate cause" of injury, then negligence has been established. In other words, the defendant's actions must bear a substantial causative relationship to the harm done.

The fourth element of a "cause of action" or lawsuit for malpractice for negligence is the actual showing of damages. For the breast interventional radiologist, this may include an unreasonable complication of a procedure, a procedure causing a delay in the diagnosis of cancer or unreasonable surgery, or improper informed consent.

Legally, therefore, it is the duty of the interventional radiologist to perform a procedure in a reasonable manner. Failure to do so, if it bears a causative relationship to some form of injury, may be the subject of a lawsuit in negligence.

The three areas of negligence that concern the breast interventional radiologist include the performance of the procedure itself, the obtaining of consent for the procedure, and the responsibility for follow-up communication and recommendations for management that involve the patient, radiologist, and referring physician.

Competency in the performance of a procedure is difficult to measure. Clinical studies often attempt to help establish the anticipated time course for developing sufficient skill of a "reasonable radiologist under similar circumstances." Presumably, skills obtained during residency may lend themselves to different circumstances so that the acquisition of new skills or modification of old ones may be facilitated by additional tutorials, continuing education courses, and even short fellowships.

Establishing competency in a new procedure to the satisfaction of anyone challenging such skill, as may occur after an adverse event, is an important component of risk management. Where conduct is suspect, documentation of prior experience, education, and familiarity with the parameters of widespread clinical trials form the basis of such a position. In addition, early experience may be accompanied by informed consent, which includes disclosure to the patient of the new incorporation of such procedures into regular clinical practice.

Stereotaxic procedures may require additional competency beyond mammographic and other image interpretation. Because the placement of a needle must be performed from one projection only, it is essential to determine that the lesion, in fact, is real and not a summation artifact. In this respect, as in any surgical procedure, selection of patients is an important component of the procedure itself. Lawsuits have been instigated for unnecessary surgery or surgery not justified by the clinical situation.[11] As stereotactic procedures increase in frequency, the importance of patient selection will increase for lesions that have been sufficiently evaluated by conventional imaging and documented as real in two orthogonal projections. Although exceptions clearly exist where the presence of a lesion is virtually unequivocal despite visualization in only one projection, such cases are rare and full work-up of orthogonal projections should be undertaken before biopsy is performed. Indeed, cases may arise for the infliction of mental distress when surgery (or perhaps stereotaxic biopsy) is recommended for indications that are not easily defensible.[12] It should be noted that such cases are unusual.

Patient selection is also an important factor in evaluating specific lesions, some of which—by experience and clinical trials—may be more prone to false-negative results. Such aspects are usually included in the obtaining of informed consent.

Success is not guaranteed in any procedure, and the law of negligence does not require a favorable result. As discussed earlier, the law evaluates conduct, not outcome. The occurrence of complications is a risk of any invasive procedure and is discussed when informed consent is obtained. As part of this process and even before, a deliberate plan should be in place to resolve a complication, if it occurs. This planning needs to include the person responsible for treating the complication and often the procedures to be followed, if such a complication occurs.

Many interventionalists are both better trained and suited to treat complications secondary to radiology procedures. Where this is not the case, it is especially important to establish an understanding among the radiologist, patient, and referring clinician regarding the appropriate transfer of care to resolve complications. Frequently, such situations are taken for granted, but the absence of a deliberate plan in the case of an untoward event may invite serious results. For example, the diagnosis and monitoring or treatment of pneumothorax after a needle that has been inserted into the breast enters the pleura may be remedied easily, but also may result in serious complications if further care is not provided. Although serious occurrences may be unlikely, a reconsideration of Judge Learned Hand's approach discussed earlier in this chapter requires an appropriate response. Understandings or even protocols developed and agreed to by participating treating physicians usually provide an adequate mechanism for such response.

LAW OF NEGLIGENCE: INFORMED CONSENT

Simple consent, appropriately obtained, is a defense to battery. Most lawsuits involving consent are not instigated for battery, but rather for the negligent obtaining of informed consent, and are thus evaluated as part of the law of negligence. It is the duty of the radiologist to obtain a reasonable consent from the patient; with respect to elective interventional procedures, this usually means informed consent.

Informed consent, unlike simple consent for battery, may require expert testimony and is a more difficult concept to understand. Informed consent has been classically defined by a federal appellate court as the disclosure of material risks and complications and alternatives available.[13] This definition is a derivative of the formula expressed previously by Judge Learned Hand, where the standard of care regarding disclosure may be seen as a determination of the product of the severity and incidence of complications. Thus any serious complications or any mild complications with high frequency should be disclosed.

Disclosure is assessed differently, depending on state jurisdiction. Several states maintain a "reasonable patient" standard such that compliance with proper consent is judged by what a reasonable patient would expect to know. Other states use a reasonable physician standard, evaluating proper consent by measuring the parameters of what a reasonable physician would disclose.[9] These nuances may have a determining influence on the final disposition of any given case, and radiologists should familiarize themselves with their own state requirements in formulating an approach to obtaining informed consent. The patient standard emphasizes more disclosure, an approach that may be preferred if, for any given set of circumstances, the physician is in doubt regarding the disclosure of a risk, regardless of the jurisdiction.

The manner of disclosure is important to avoid unnecessary anxiety and potentially adverse effects of a patient refusing an important procedure. The approach requires a balance, and sometimes finesse, in disclosing risks clearly without incurring undue fear. The difficulty of such an approach is evidenced by one published report indicating that 121 of 1513

(8 percent) radiologists surveyed have been involved with informed consent litigation.[14]

Much attention has been paid to the production of a proper informed consent form. Certainly, procedure-specific forms are preferred, but are not often necessary. Obtaining informed consent is a process, and emphasis needs to be placed on a meaningful discussion between the physician performing the procedure and the patient. The written consent form is simply evidence of such a discussion, nothing more or less. Thus, the signed consent form is not synonymous with informed consent and is, in fact, subordinate to the discussion. A regular and repetitive recitation of known risks, best validated by a protocol and witnessed by other persons, is the essence of the process. Together with a signed form, a factual basis for reasonable conduct is thus established. Informed consent often requires disclosure of alternatives and occasionally the consequences of not undergoing the procedure. Although exceptions occur to the obtaining of informed consent, they are generally not applicable to elective interventional breast procedures.

The person performing the procedure must obtain the consent. Residents, colleagues, or other personnel may not substitute for the person doing the procedure. Often, details of the procedure may be related by other providers so that the discussion time is shortened between the interventionalist and the patient. This approach is permissible, so long as the essence of the consent is obtained by the physician involved. Tissue sampling and preoperative localizations by image guidance require an additional consideration in obtaining informed consent. As has been documented in clinical studies, tissue sampling procedures with failed surgical attempts are associated with a finite percentage of nondiagnostic yields and preoperative localizations.[15,16] Disclosure of these possibilities is an important component of the consent process. Because such circumstances are unusual but do occur, informed consent requires a consideration of their occurrence.

THE LAW OF NEGLIGENCE: REASONABLE MANAGEMENT

Radiologists have for some time been involved with image-guided tissue sampling. Fine needle aspiration of pancreatic or hepatic lesions in hospitalized patients has become part of regular clinical practice, frequently without appropriate protocols. In fact, a "closed loop" situation regarding results and communication is predicated on the nature of the inpatient setting, as is accountability in the form of quality assurance and peer review required by the Joint Commission on the Accreditation of Health Organizations.

The issue of tissue sampling and deliberate planning becomes more difficult for the breast interventionalist, where most procedures are performed on an outpatient basis and, therefore, lack many of the previously mentioned internal controls that pre-empt untoward events. A reconsideration of fundamental aspects of such procedures, therefore, is important.

State courts vary in their view of the radiologist in patient care. In California, for example, a radiologist's role is defined as a consultant, with the state's highest court indicating that interference with the clinician-patient relationship may invite unnecessary problems.[17] Other courts have taken different views; in fact, the relationship of patients to interventional radiologists, in many circumstances, may be evolving. Thus, universal solutions to such problems do not exist. Unfortunately, some "experts" often insist that one approach is not only favorable but required to meet the standard of care, a misleading position that has been criticized.[2] Fundamentally, if a primary care physician refers a patient to a radiologist for an interventional procedure, reports should be directed to the referring clinician. In fact, this approach for breast interventional procedures is in keeping with the logic of the MQSA. Aspects of patient notification may be subject to further regulatory directives.

Different circumstances require the interventional radiologist to define his or her specific role. When there are no other treating physicians, pathology results need to be sent directly to the radiologist. In such a situation, the radiologist is the primary provider for the patient and is responsible for relating the results and consequent management recommendations to the patient. When the radiologist serves a consultative role, he or she may still desire a copy of the results to be sent to the imaging facility, in addition to the primary treating physician. In such circumstances, the treating physician is still considered the "ordering" physician and should expect the results to be forthcoming, as in the ordering of any test. Optimal patient management is facilitated when the interventional radiologist confirms and/or discusses the results with the ordering physician. Where results have not or cannot be communicated by the referring physician to the patient—extraordinary circumstances that should be documented—results may need to be communicated either directly to the patient or, with proper transfer of care for the patient, to another clinician agreeing to assume responsibility for patient management. This "default" responsibility follows from the foreseeable consequences known to the radiologist participating in the biopsy on an outpatient basis: namely, if a malignant diagnosis is not otherwise communicated to the patient, untoward consequences will occur. In this manner, the initially subordinate role of the consulting radiologist is elevated to a primary role, dictated by circumstances for which contingency planning should be established.

Breast imaging occupies an unusual role in radiology in that patients who have no other physician may self-refer themselves to a given imaging facility. Such facilities extend their role to that of primary care providers.[18,19] When interventional procedures are then undertaken, the role of primary care provider requires that the radiologist provide the patient directly with the results of the test, including that of tissue sampling. Furthermore, if additional surgery is required, appropriate referral and transfer of care are required as part of the standard of care. Mechanisms should be instituted to verify either compliance with such recommendations for referral, or documented efforts to achieve compliance.

Special communication problems may be anticipated by the public health nature of breast imaging and screening mammography. Whereas most radiologic consultations are prompted by signs or symptoms of disease, causing a patient to seek clinical evaluation for which subsequent radiologic examinations are performed, healthy women under the care of a primary physician may "self-initiate" a mammographic study. This practice should be distinguished from self-referral, a situation reserved for women not under the care of another physician. When such screening-detected abnormalities lead to on-site immediate tissue sampling or other procedures, communication and management problems may arise. This is especially true when the patient requests such tissue sampling, placing the radiologist in a role of primary responsibility for which he or she is unaccustomed, because the primary care

physician has been bypassed, if he or she has not been consulted about the performance of a biopsy. One approach to this dilemma is for the radiologist to discuss the case with the primary physician before performing further interventions.

It is of paramount concern that a designated physician be responsible for communicating results and issuing management recommendations to the patient in a manner designed for both patient compliance and subsequent follow-up care. As mentioned, custom has conferred this responsibility on the clinician, with the radiologist serving as a consultant. Modifications of this system that achieve the same goals and conform to similar standards of care are permissible and may even be encouraged, depending on the circumstances surrounding patient care.

THE LAW OF NEGLIGENCE: DERIVATIVE TORTS

The interventional breast radiologist should be familiar with still other civil actions or "torts." These are based on the more primary aspects of care rendered; therefore, these issues have been reserved traditionally for the clinical community. If they perform interventional procedures, however, they will now affect radiologists.[20]

The tort of "abandonment" arises when the care of a patient either suffering a complication of a procedure or receiving results that require further care (e.g., surgery) are not resolved by the primary care provider, which may be the radiologist. The transfer of care to another provider may be a required aspect of the interventional radiologist in fulfilling the standard of care. The extent to which the radiologist must go in transferring such care depends on the exigencies and severity of the circumstances. For more serious situations, adequate documentation is important, particularly if the patient chooses to decline recommendations.

Another tort called "negligent referral" occurs when a physician refers a patient to another treating physician or facility, which he or she knows or has reason to know is not suitably competent to resolve a medical situation, and an untoward event occurs. Not only is the treating physician exposed to legal redress for such an untoward event, but the referring physician is also exposed to a lawsuit for "negligent referral." In the past, radiologists serving as consultants have not usually been in a position to make direct referrals. With the advent of both self-referral and self-initiated mammograms prompting subsequent procedures and interventions, however, radiologists may find themselves in a position to refer patients for further treatment. Such referral, as for all conduct subject to the tort of negligence, needs to be reasonable.

SUMMARY

Data regarding lawsuits against radiologists may vary, depending on whether the information is derived from settlement of claims, data, trial data, or appellate court data. Each of these analyses is compromised by certain design biases. Virtually all large studies indicate a rising number of malpractice lawsuits against radiologists in general. Combined with the increased exposure from those involved in interventional procedures and those involved with breast disease evaluation, such legal exposure should prompt caution, but not alarm. An understanding of the legal parameters regarding breast interventional procedures and a deliberate appropriate approach to such circumstances should provide those involved in this exciting field with a basis for both defeating unfounded claims and discouraging future ones.

REFERENCES

1. Physicians Association of America. Breast Cancer Study of 1995. Physicians Association of America. Washington, DC, 1995.
2. Brenner RJ. Mammography and malpractice litigation: current status, lessons, and admonitions. Am J Roentgenol 1993; 161:931–935.
2a. Cyrak D. Induced costs of low-cost screening mammography. Radiology 1988; 168:661–664.
3. Texas Medical Association. Medical professional liability: an examination of claims frequency and severity in Texas. Texas Medical Association, Tonn & Associates. Houston, TX, 1994
4. Bowyer EA. High radiology losses related to invasive procedures. Risk Management Foundation Forum 1985; 6:1–8.
5. McCormick B. Don't criminalize medical judgment. Am Med News 1993; 36:6.
6. Mammography Quality Standards Act of 1972, PL 102–539.
7. Reynolds HE, Jackson VP, Musick BS. A survey of interventional mammography practices. Radiology 1993; 187:71–73.
8. Brenner RJ, Eth S, Trygstad CW. Defining the risks of venipuncture(letter). N Engl J Med 1976; 295:53–54.
9. Reuter SR. An overview of informed consent for radiologists. Am J Roentgenol 1987; 148:219–227.
10. Restatement(second) of Torts, Section 323(a).
11. *Kinikin v Heupel*, 305 NW2d 589 (1981).
12. *Hume v Bayer*, 178 NJ Super 370, 428 A2d 961 (NJ 1981).
13. *Cantebury v Spence*, 464 F2d 772 (DC Cir (1972).
14. Hamer MM, Morlock F, Foley HT et al. Medical malpractice in diagnostic radiology: claims, compensation, and patient injury. Radiology 1987; 164:263–266.
15. Brenner RJ, Bassett LW, Dershaw DD et al. Percutaneous core biopsy of the breast: a multisite prospective trial. Radiology 1994; 193(P):295.
16. Homer MJ, Smith TJ, Safaii H. Prebiopsy needle localization: methods, problems, and expected results. Radiol Clin North Am 1992; 30:139–154.
17. *Townsend v Turk*, 266 Cal App 3d 278, 1266 Cal Rptr 821 (1990).
18. Monsees B, Destouet JM, Evens RG. The self-referred mammography patient: a new responsibility for radiologists. Radiology 1988; 166:69–71.
19. Brenner RJ. Medicolegal aspects of breast imaging: variable standards of care relating to different types of practice. Am J Roentgenol 1991; 156:719–723.
20. Brenner RJ. Breast cancer evaluation: medical-legal and risk management considerations for the clinician. Cancer (suppl) 1994; 74:486–491.

INDEX

Page numbers followed by f *represent figures; those followed by* t *represent tables*